Year Book of Dermatology – 2019
ACNE

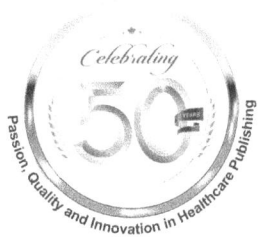

Year Book of Dermatology – 2019
ACNE

Editors

Shashi Kumar BM MD (DVL) FIADVL (Dermatopath)
Associate Professor
Department of Dermatology
Mandya Institute of Medical Sciences
Mandya, Karnataka, India

Savitha AS MD (DVL) DNB FRGUHS (Dermatosurgery)
Associate Professor
Department of Dermatology
Sapthagiri Institute of Medical Science and Research Center
Bengaluru, Karnataka, India

R Raghunatha Reddy MD (DVL) DNB FRGUHS (Dermatosurgery)
Professor and Head
Department of Dermatology
Akash Institute of Medical Sciences and Research Centre
Bengaluru, Karnataka, India

Foreword
Ramesh Bhat M MD

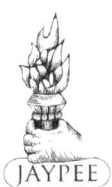

JAYPEE BROTHERS MEDICAL PUBLISHERS
The Health Sciences Publisher
New Delhi | London

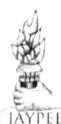 **Jaypee Brothers Medical Publishers (P) Ltd**

Headquarters
Jaypee Brothers Medical Publishers (P) Ltd
4838/24, Ansari Road, Daryaganj
New Delhi 110 002, India
Phone: +91-11-43574357
Fax: +91-11-43574314
Email: jaypee@jaypeebrothers.com

Overseas Offices
J.P. Medical Ltd
83 Victoria Street, London
SW1H 0HW (UK)
Phone: +44 20 3170 8910
Fax: +44 (0)20 3008 6180
Email: info@jpmedpub.com

Website: www.jaypeebrothers.com
Website: www.jaypeedigital.com

© 2019, Jaypee Brothers Medical Publishers

The views and opinions expressed in this book are solely those of the original contributor(s)/author(s) and do not necessarily represent those of editor(s) of the book.

All rights reserved. No part of this publication may be reproduced, stored or transmitted in any form or by any means, electronic, mechanical, photocopying, recording or otherwise, without the prior permission in writing of the publishers.

All brand names and product names used in this book are trade names, service marks, trademarks or registered trademarks of their respective owners. The publisher is not associated with any product or vendor mentioned in this book.

Medical knowledge and practice change constantly. This book is designed to provide accurate, authoritative information about the subject matter in question. However, readers are advised to check the most current information available on procedures included and check information from the manufacturer of each product to be administered, to verify the recommended dose, formula, method and duration of administration, adverse effects and contraindications. It is the responsibility of the practitioner to take all appropriate safety precautions. Neither the publisher nor the author(s)/editor(s) assume any liability for any injury and/or damage to persons or property arising from or related to use of material in this book.

This book is sold on the understanding that the publisher is not engaged in providing professional medical services. If such advice or services are required, the services of a competent medical professional should be sought.

Every effort has been made where necessary to contact holders of copyright to obtain permission to reproduce copyright material. If any have been inadvertently overlooked, the publisher will be pleased to make the necessary arrangements at the first opportunity. The **CD/DVD-ROM** (if any) provided in the sealed envelope with this book is complimentary and free of cost. **Not meant for sale.**

Inquiries for bulk sales may be solicited at: jaypee@jaypeebrothers.com

Year Book of Dermatology – 2019 *Acne* / Shashi Kumar BM, Savitha AS, R Raghunatha Reddy

First Edition: **2019**

ISBN: 978-93-89188-49-3

Dedicated to

*All our friends
who have contributed to this book.*

CONTRIBUTORS

Editors

Shashi Kumar BM MD (DVL) FIADVL (Dermatopath)
Associate Professor
Department of Dermatology
Mandya Institute of Medical Sciences
Mandya, Karnataka, India

Savitha AS MD (DVL) DNB FRGUHS (Dermatosurgery)
Associate Professor
Department of Dermatology
Sapthagiri Institute of Medical Science and Research Center
Bengaluru, Karnataka, India

R Raghunatha Reddy MD (DVL) DNB FRGUHS (Dermatosurgery)
Professor and Head
Department of Dermatology
Akash Institute of Medical Sciences and Research Centre
Bengaluru, Karnataka, India

Contributing Authors

Eshwari L MD RGUHS (Dermatosurgery)
Assistant Professor
Bangalore Medical College and Research Centre
Bengaluru, Karnataka, India

Lakshmi DV DVD
Senior Resident
Bangalore Medical College and Research Centre
Bengaluru, Karnataka, India

Madura C MD RGUHS (Dermatosurgery)
Consultant Dermatologist
CUTIS Academy of Cutaneous Sciences
Bengaluru, Karnataka, India

Nagesh TS MD (DVL) DNB
Professor and Head
Department of Dermatology, Sapthagiri Institute of Medical Science and Research Center
Bengaluru, Karnataka, India

Shilpa K MD RGUHS (Dermatosurgery)
Assistant Professor
Bangalore Medical College and Research Centre
Bengaluru, Karnataka, India

Sneha M MD (DVL)
Senior Resident, Department of Dermatology
Sapthagiri Institute of Medical Science and Research Centre
Bengaluru, Karnataka, India

FOREWORD

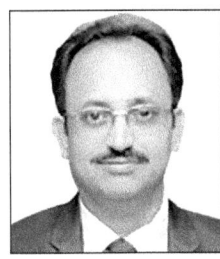

Ramesh Bhat M MD
Director, ILDS
President, IADVL (National)–2018
Professor, Father Muller Medical College
Kankanady, Mangaluru, Karnataka, India
Former Hon. General Secretary IADVL (National 2010–12)

Acne is a skin disease which affects almost everybody at sometime during the lifetime. With more affluent concepts of living, this condition has become routinely seen in pre and post adolescent age group also. In view of the multiple etiopathogenic factors, we have many a treatment modalities also.

Acne is an important and preferred area of research by Dermatologists and Pharma industry. We see many a publications in this field particularly in areas of Etiopathogenesis, Quality of life and Treatment modalities. Sometimes it's very difficult to gather all the recent advances in the field of management of this common problem.

The *Year Book of Dermatology – 2019 Acne* has the advantage of compilation of all the recent advances in the field of Acne. The Editors have not only compiled various research articles but also have given key messages and expert comments. This will help not only practitioners but also researchers and postgraduate residents.

Hereby, I congratulate Dr Shashi Kumar BM, Dr Savitha AS, the ever hardworking and enthusiastic young dermatologists ably guided and inspired by R Raghunatha Reddy.

I am sure that, this book will be welcomed by Dermatologists with enthusiasm and eagerness.

I sincerely thank the trio of editors and wish them all the best.

PREFACE

Acne is the most common dermatological condition with profound morbidity. Understanding of causes and contributory factors has taken major steps forward over the past few years. There is an increasing knowledge about acne pathogenesis which has led to newer insight to therapies. This year book on acne has collection of original abstracts of path breaking research published in high impact factor journals that were published in the previous year. It presents breakthrough developments articles which were reviewed thoroughly and commented on the value of the article.

Shashi Kumar BM
Savitha AS
R Raghunatha Reddy

CONTENTS

1. Treatment of Moderate Acne Vulgaris in Fitzpatrick Skin Type V or VI: Efficacy and Tolerability of Fixed Combination Clindamycin Phosphate 1.2%/Benzoyl Peroxide 3.75% Gel 1

2. Novel Tretinoin 0.05% Lotion for the Once-daily Treatment of Moderate-to-severe Acne Vulgaris: Assessment of Efficacy and Safety in Patients aged 9 Years and Older 2

3. Once-daily Oral Sarecycline 1.5 mg/kg/day is Effective for Moderate-to-severe Acne Vulgaris: Results from Two Identically Designed, Phase 3, Randomized, Double-blind Clinical Trials 3

4. The Efficacy and Safety of Azelaic Acid 15% Foam in the Treatment of Facial Acne Vulgaris 4

5. Frequency of Treatment Switching for Spironolactone Compared to Oral Tetracycline-class Antibiotics for Women with Acne: A Retrospective Cohort Study 2010–2016 5

6. Clinical Experience with Once-daily Dapsone Gel, 7.5% Monotherapy in Patients with Acne Vulgaris 7

7. An Acne Survey from the World's Largest Annual Gathering of Twins 8

8. Efficacy and Safety of Adapalene 0.3%/Benzoyl Peroxide 2.5% Gel plus Oral Doxycycline in Subjects with Severe Inflammatory Acne who are Candidates for Oral Isotretinoin 9

9. Efficacy, Safety and Tolerability of Topical Dapsone Gel, 7.5% for Treatment of Acne Vulgaris by Fitzpatrick Skin Phototype 10

10. Clinical Significance of Neutrophil Gelatinase-associated Lipocalin and Galectin-7 in Tape-stripped Stratum Corneum of Acne Vulgaris 11

11. Risk of Depression among Patients with Acne: A Population-based Cohort Study using The Health Improvement Network (THIN) Database 12

12. Acne Development in Male Androgenetic Alopecia 13

13. Effects of Isotretinoin Treatment on Affective and Cognitive Functions in Adolescent Acne Vulgaris Patients 14

14. Analysis of Gut Microbiome in Patients with Acne Vulgaris 15

15. Isotretinoin Therapy: A Retrospective Cohort Analysis of Completion Rates and Factors Associated with Nonadherence 16

16. Photodynamic Therapy for Acne Conglobata of the Buttocks: Effective Anti-inflammatory Treatment with Good Cosmetic Outcome — 17

17. Acneiform Eruptions: An Unusual Dermatological Side Effect of Ribavirin — 18

18. Topical Dapsone Gel is a New Treatment Option for Acne Agminata — 19

19. The Effect of Continuous High versus Low Dose Oral Isotretinoin Regimens on Dermcidin Expression in Patients with Moderate-to-severe Acne Vulgaris — 20

20. Transgender Adolescents and Acne: A Case Series — 21

21. Chemical Peels in the Treatment of Acne: Patient Selection and Perspectives — 22

22. A Novel Cognitive Stress Management Technique for Acne Vulgaris: A Short Report of a Pilot Experimental Study — 24

23. Evaluation of the Efficacy of Microneedle Fractional Radiofrequency in Turkish Patients with Atrophic Facial Acne Scars — 25

24. Effect of Oral Isotretinoin on the Nucleocytoplasmic Distribution of FoxO1 and FoxO3 Proteins in Sebaceous Glands of Patients with Acne Vulgaris — 27

25. Adult-onset Acne: Prevalence, Impact and Management Challenges — 29

26. Acne: A Side Effect of Masculinizing Hormonal Therapy in Transgender Patients — 31

27. Efficacy and Safety Profile of Spironolactone 50 mg v/s Isotretinoin 10 mg in the Treatment of Female Patients with Acne Vulgaris Grade 1-2—A Double Blinded, Randomized Comparative Study — 32

28. The Microbiome in Preadolescent Acne: Assessment and Prospective Analysis of the Influence of Benzoyl Peroxide — 34

29. Association of Systemic Antibiotic Treatment of Acne with Skin Microbiota Characteristics — 35

30. Novel Nicotinamide Skin-adhesive Hot Melt Extrudates for Treatment of Acne — 36

31. Treatment of Acne with a Combination of Propolis, Tea Tree Oil and *Aloe vera* Compared to Erythromycin Cream: Two Double-blind Investigations — 38

32. The Safety and Efficacy of Four Different Fixed Combination Regimens of Adapalene 0.1%/Benzoyl Peroxide 2.5% Gel for the Treatment of Acne Vulgaris: Results from a Randomized Controlled Study — 39

33. Survey of Acne-related Post-inflammatory Hyperpigmentation in the Middle East — 41

34. The Use of Hormonal Antiandrogen Therapy in Female Patients with Acne: A 10-year Retrospective Study — 42

35. Adapalene 0.3% Gel Shows Efficacy for the Treatment of Atrophic Acne Scars — 43

36. Evaluation the Efficacy of Trichloroacetic Acid 33% in Treatment of Oral Retinoid-induced Cheilitis Compared with Placebo (Vaseline): A Randomized Pilot Study — 45

37. Light Therapies for Acne: Abridged Cochrane Systematic Review including GRADE Assessments — 46

38. Dapsone-loaded Invasomes as a Potential Treatment of Acne: Preparation, Characterization and In Vivo Skin Deposition Assay — 48

39. Prevention and Reduction of Atrophic Acne Scars with Adapalene 0.3%/Benzoyl Peroxide 2.5% Gel in Subjects with Moderate or Severe Facial Acne: Results of a 6-month Randomized, Vehicle-controlled Trial using Intra-individual Comparison — 49

40. Complementary and Alternative Methods for Treatment of Acne Vulgaris: A Systematic Review — 50

41. Effects of the Myrtle Essential Oil on the Acne Skin—Clinical Trials for Korean Women — 52

42. Comparison of Efficacy of Commercially Available versus Freshly Prepared Salicylic Acid Peel in Treatment of Acne: A Randomized Open-label Study — 53

43. A Comparison of Combined Oral Contraceptives Containing Chlormadinone Acetate versus Drospirenone for the Treatment of Acne and Dysmenorrhea: A Randomized Trial — 54

44. Efficacy and Adverse Events of Oral Isotretinoin for Acne: A Systematic Review — 56

45. Aromatherapy, Botanicals, and Essential Oils in Acne — 58

46. A Review of Diagnosis and Treatment of Acne in Adult Female Patients — 59

47. Clinical Evidence for Washing and Cleansers in Acne Vulgaris: A Systematic Review — 60

48. ROS-responsive Microneedle Patch for Acne Vulgaris Treatment — 62

49. Optimizing the Use of Topical Retinoids in Asian Acne Patients — 63

50. Comparative Study of the Efficacy of Platelet-rich Plasma Combined with Carboxytherapy versus its Use with Fractional Carbon Dioxide Laser in Atrophic Acne Scars — 64

51. Effects of Oral Supplementation with FOS and GOS Prebiotics in Women with Adult Acne: The "SO Sweet" Study: A Proof-of-concept Pilot Trial — 66

52. Approaches to Limit Systemic Antibiotic Use in Acne: Systemic Alternatives, Emerging Topical Therapies, Dietary Modification, and Laser and Light-based Treatments — 67

53. The Efficacy and Tolerability of 5-aminolevulinic Acid 5% Thermosetting Gel Photodynamic Therapy in the Treatment of Mild-to-moderate Acne Vulgaris. A Two-center, Prospective Assessor-blinded, Proof-of-concept Study — 69

54. Combination Chemical Peels are More Effective than Single Chemical Peel in Treatment of Mild-to-moderate Acne Vulgaris: A Split Face Comparative Clinical Trial ... 70

55. Comparison of Efficacy of Aminolevulinic Acid Photodynamic Therapy versus Adapalene Gel plus Oral Doxycycline for Treatment of Moderate Acne Vulgaris – A Simple, Blind, Randomized, and Controlled Trial ... 72

56. Microneedling by Dermapen and Glycolic Acid Peel for the Treatment of Acne Scars: Comparative Study ... 73

57. Antipruritic Efficacies of Doxycycline and Erythromycin in the Treatment of Acne Vulgaris: A Randomized Single-blinded Pilot Study ... 75

58. Does Isotretinoin Cause Depression and Anxiety in Acne Patients? ... 76

59. Treatment of Atrophic Acne Scarring with Fractional Micro-plasma Radiofrequency in Chinese Patients: A Prospective Study ... 78

60. Comparison of Novel Dual Mode versus Conventional Single Pass of a 1450-nm Diode Laser in the Treatment of Acne Vulgaris for Korean Patients: A 20-week Prospective, Randomized, Split-face Study ... 80

61. Resurfacing of Facial Acne Scars with a New Variable-pulsed Er:YAG Laser in Fitzpatrick Skin Types IV and V ... 82

62. A Novel Topical Minocycline Foam for the Treatment of Moderate-to-severe Acne Vulgaris: Results of 2 Randomized, Double-blind, Phase 3 Studies ... 83

63. Management of Comedonal Acne Vulgaris with Fixed-combination Topical Therapy ... 85

64. Blunt Cannula Subcision is more Effective than Nokor Needle Subcision for Acne Scars Treatment ... 86

65. Novel Tretinoin 0.05% Lotion for the Once-daily Treatment of Moderate-to-severe Acne Vulgaris in a Preadolescent Population ... 88

66. Efficacy of Two Plant Extracts Against Acne Vulgaris: Initial Results of Microbiological Tests and Cell Culture Studies ... 90

67. Female Type of Adult Acne: Physiological and Psychological Considerations and Management ... 91

68. The Efficacy and Safety of Nonpharmacological Therapies for the Treatment of Acne Vulgaris: A Systematic Review and Best-evidence Synthesis ... 94

69. Clindamycin Phosphate 1.2%/Benzoyl Peroxide 3% Fixed-dose Combination Gel versus Topical Combination Therapy of Adapalene 0.1% Gel and Clindamycin Phosphate 1.2% Gel in the Treatment of Acne Vulgaris in Japanese Patients: A Multicenter, Randomized, Investigator-blind, Parallel-group Study ... 96

70. Screening of Body Dysmorphic Disorder in Acne Patients: A Pilot Study	97
71. A Qualitative Investigation of the Impact of Acne on Health-related Quality of Life: Development of a Conceptual Model	99
72. Host-microbiome Interactions and Recent Progress into Understanding the Biology of Acne Vulgaris	100
73. Acne in Lomé, Togo: Clinical Aspects and Quality of Life of Patients	102
74. The Role of the Physician in Patient Perceptions of Barriers to Primary Adherence with Acne Medications	103
75. Exploring the Relationship between Stress and Acne: A Medical Student's Perspective	105
76. The Impact of Acne and Facial Postinflammatory Hyperpigmentation on Quality of Life and Self-esteem of Newly Admitted Nigerian Undergraduates	106
77. Which Acne Treatment has the Best Influence on Health-related Quality of Life? Literature Review by the European Academy of Dermatology and Venereology Task Force on Quality of Life and Patient Oriented Outcomes	107
78. Stressful Life Events and Psychiatric Comorbidity in Acne–A Case Control Study	109
79. The Evaluation of Psychiatric Comorbidity, Self-injurious Behavior, Suicide Probability, and other Associated Psychiatric Factors (Loneliness, Self-esteem, Life Satisfaction) in Adolescents with Acne: A Clinical Pilot Study	111
80. Acne Relapses: Impact on Quality of Life and Productivity	112
81. The Mental Health Burden in Acne Vulgaris and Rosacea: An Analysis of the US National Inpatient Sample	113
82. The Therapeutic Effect of Tanshinone IIA on *Propionibacterium acnes*-induced Inflammation In Vitro	115
83. Anti-acne Properties of Hydrophobic Fraction of Red Ginseng (Panax Ginseng C.A. Meyer) and its Active Components	116
84. Mechanistic Insight into the Activity of a Sulfone Compound Dapsone on *Propionibacterium* (Newly Reclassified as *Cutibacterium*) Acnes–mediated Cytokine Production	118
85. Lipidomics Reveals Skin Surface Lipid Abnormity in Male Youth Acne	120
86. Acne Vulgaris Severity Graded by In Vivo Reflectance Confocal Microscopy and Optical Coherence Tomography	121
87. Vitamin D Levels in Acne Vulgaris Patients Treated with Oral Isotretinoin	124
88. The Effect of Milk Consumption on Acne: A Meta-analysis of Observational Studies	125

89. Acne and Nutrition: Hypotheses, Myths and Facts — 127

90. Enhancement of Lipid Content and Inflammatory Cytokine Secretion in SZ95 Sebocytes by Palmitic Acid Suggests a Potential Link between Free Fatty Acids and Acne Aggravation — 129

91. Characterization of *Cutibacterium acnes* Phylotypes in Acne and In Vivo Exploratory Evaluation of Myrtacine — 130

92. Atrophic Scar Formation in Acne Patients involves Long-acting Immune Responses with Plasma Cells and Alteration of Sebaceous Gland — 132

93. Lesional and Circulating Levels of Interleukin-17 and 25 Hydroxy-cholecalciferol in Active Acne Vulgaris: Correlation to Disease Severity — 134

94. Clinical Efficacy of 0.5% Topical Mangosteen Extract in Nanoparticle Loaded Gel in Treatment of Mild-to-moderate Acne Vulgaris: A 12-Week, Split-Face, Double-blinded, Randomized, Controlled Trial — 136

95. The Influence of Exposome on Acne — 138

96. Association of Interleukin-6 Gene Promoter Polymorphism with Acne Vulgaris and its Severity — 139

97. Genome-wide Meta-analysis Implicates Mediators of Hair Follicle Development and Morphogenesis in Risk for Severe Acne — 141

98. Microbiological Profile of Sarecycline: A Novel Targeted Spectrum Tetracycline for the Treatment of Acne Vulgaris — 143

99. Daily Intake of Soft Drinks and Moderate-to-severe Acne Vulgaris in Chinese Adolescents — 144

100. New Concepts, Concerns, and Creations in Acne — 146

101. The Anti-inflammatory Activities of *Propionibacterium acnes* CAMP Factor-targeted Acne Vaccines — 148

102. Skin Ecology during Sebaceous Drought—How Skin Microbes Respond to Isotretinoin — 149

103. *Propionibacterium acnes*-derived Extracellular Vesicles Promote Acne-like Phenotypes in Human Epidermis — 150

104. Patients with Acne Vulgaris have a Distinct Gut Microbiota in Comparison with Healthy Controls — 152

105. Inhibitory Effects of *Euphorbia supina* on *Propionibacterium acnes*-induced Skin Inflammation In Vitro and In Vivo — 153

106. Isolation and Identification of the Follicular Microbiome: Implications for Acne Research — 154

107.	Expression of Inflammatory and Fibrogenetic Markers in Acne Hypertrophic Scar Formation: Focusing on Role of TGF-β and IGF-1R	156
108.	Decrease in Diversity of *Propionibacterium acnes* Phylotypes in Patients with Severe Acne on the Back	158
109.	Short Lipopeptides Specifically Inhibit the Growth of *Propionibacterium acnes* with Antibacterial and Anti-inflammatory Dual Action	159
110.	Plasma Exeresis for Active Acne Vulgaris: Clinical and In Vivo Microscopic Documentation of Treatment Efficacy by Means of Reflectance Confocal Microscopy	161
111.	Licochalcone A Attenuates Acne Symptoms Mediated by Suppression of NLRP3 Inflammasome	162
112.	Gut Microbiota Alterations in Moderate-to-severe Acne Vulgaris Patients	163
113.	Overall and Subgroup Prevalence of Acne Vulgaris among Patients with Hidradenitis Suppurativa	164
114.	Association of the TNF-α Gene Promoter Polymorphisms at Nucleotide-238 and -308 with Acne Susceptibility: A Meta-analysis	166
115.	Tumor Necrosis Factor α-308 G/A and Interleukin 1 β-511 C/T Gene Polymorphisms in Patients with Scarring Acne	167
116.	SIG1459: A Novel Phytyl-Cysteine Derived TLR2 Modulator with In Vitro and Clinical Anti-acne Activity	169
117.	Associations among Two Vitamin D Receptor (VDR) Gene Polymorphisms (ApaI and TaqI) in Acne Vulgaris: A Pilot Susceptibility Study	170
118.	Using Network Oriented Research Assistant (NORA) Technology to Compare Digital Photographic with In-Person Assessment of Acne Vulgaris	172
119.	Genetic Association between the *NLRP3* Gene and Acne Vulgaris in a Chinese Population	173
120.	Serum Irisin: A Prognostic Marker for Severe Acne Vulgaris	175
121.	Primary Sebocytes and Sebaceous Gland Cell Lines for Studying Sebaceous Lipogenesis and Sebaceous Gland Diseases	178
122.	Acne Vulgaris in Patients with Hidradenitis Suppurativa	180
123.	Validation of 3D Skin Imaging for Objective Repeatable Quantification of Severity of Atrophic Acne Scarring	181
124.	No Evidence for Follicular Keratinocyte Hyperproliferation in Acne Lesions as Compared to Autologous Healthy Hair Follicles	183

125. Seasonal Changes in Epidermal Ceramides are Linked to Impaired
Barrier Function in Acne Patients — 185

126. *Cutibacterium acnes (Propionibacterium acnes)* and Acne Vulgaris: A Brief Look
at the Latest Updates — 187

127. The In Vitro Antimicrobial Evaluation of Commercial Essential Oils and
their Combinations against Acne — 189

128. Seasonal Aggravation of Acne in Summers and the Effect of Temperature and
Humidity in a Study in a Tropical Setting — 192

129. Acne Prevalence in 9–14-year-old Patients Attending Pediatric
Ambulatory Clinics in Italy — 194

130. Confocal Microscopy in Adult Women with Acne — 196

131. Erythema-directed Digital Photography for the Enhanced Evaluation of
Topical Treatments for Acne Vulgaris — 198

132. Acne Vulgaris: The Metabolic Syndrome of the Pilosebaceous Follicle — 200

133. Circular RNA Expression Profile Analysis of Severe Acne by RNA-Seq
and Bioinformatics — 202

134. Taxonomy and Phylogeny of *Cutibacterium* (formerly *Propionibacterium*) *acnes* in
Inflammatory Skin Diseases — 204

135. Transforming Acne Care by Pediatricians: An Interventional Cohort Study — 205

Index — *207*

ARTICLE 1

Treatment of Moderate Acne Vulgaris in Fitzpatrick Skin Type V or VI: Efficacy and Tolerability of Fixed Combination Clindamycin Phosphate 1.2%/Benzoyl Peroxide 3.75% Gel

Amar L, Kircik LH. Treatment of Moderate Acne Vulgaris in Fitzpatrick Skin Type V or VI: Efficacy and Tolerability of Fixed Combination Clindamycin Phosphate 1.2%/Benzoyl Peroxide 3.75% Gel.
J Drugs Dermatol. 2018;17(10):1107-12.

Abstract

Acne vulgaris is a common chronic disorder of adolescence, the sequel-like scarring and pigmentation causing severe psychological distress. In US a open-label study, patients were treated with a higher concentration of the well-known fixed combination of clindamycin with benzoyl peroxide. Clindamycin phosphate 1.2%/benzoyl peroxide 3.75% gel was prescribed in 20 patients for Fitzpatrick Skin Type V or VI and with moderate facial acne once daily for 16 weeks. Significant reductions in inflammatory, noninflammatory, and total lesions occurred within the first 4 weeks compared to baseline. Additionally, Post inflammatory hyperpigmentation (PIH) severity and distribution were also significantly reduced by week 16. The combination was well tolerated.

COMMENT

Complications of acne-like scarring and hyperpigmentation are more in people of skin with color. This study was conducted in individuals with Fitzpatrick Skin Type V or VI. In an open-label study, 20 patients with moderate facial acne were treated with clindamycin phosphate 1.2%/benzoyl peroxide 3.75% gel. The application was once daily for 16 weeks. Assessment was done based on investigator global assessment of acne, postinflammatory pigmentation severity, and lesion count reduction. Side effects were also noted. Significant reductions in inflammatory, noninflammatory, and total lesions occurred within the first 4 weeks compared to baseline. Additionally, PIH severity and distribution were also significantly reduced by week 16. In 40% of patients, PIH severity was rated as "none" or "slight"; 19 (95%) of patients experienced at least a 1-grade improvement in PIH severity or distribution. About 10 patients complained of adverse events, but none were severe. There was no discontinuation of usage due to adverse events.

Key Message

- *Patients with Fitzpatrick Skin Type V and VI treated with clindamycin phosphate 1.2%/ benzoyl peroxide 3.75% gel experienced significant reductions in facial acne severity, lesion counts, and PIH severity/distribution. Tolerability was excellent.*

ARTICLE 2

Novel Tretinoin 0.05% Lotion for the Once-daily Treatment of Moderate-to-severe Acne Vulgaris: Assessment of Efficacy and Safety in Patients aged 9 Years and Older

Tyring SK, Kircik LH, Pariser DM, et al. Novel Tretinoin 0.05% Lotion for the Once-Daily Treatment of Moderate-to-Severe Acne Vulgaris: Assessment of Efficacy and Safety in Patients Aged 9 Years and Older.
J Drugs Dermatol. 2018;17(10):1084-91.

Abstract

Topical tretinoin is used extensively in noninflammatory acne vulgaris, commonly in gel and cream formulations. The objective of this study was to evaluate the efficacy, safety, and tolerability of a novel tretinoin 0.05% lotion in moderate-to-severe acne among patients aged 9 years and older. A total of 1,640 patients were randomized to receive tretinoin 0.05% lotion or vehicle for 12 weeks, and efficacy and safety of tretinoin were evaluated. Tretinoin 0.05% lotion demonstrated statistically significant superiority to vehicle in reducing inflammatory and noninflammatory lesion counts at week 12. Tretinoin 0.05% lotion also showed significantly greater benefits relative to vehicle control in terms of patient satisfaction and acne-specific quality of life domains. Tretinoin 0.05% lotion was very well tolerated with no substantive differences in cutaneous tolerability among treatment groups. No patients discontinued treatment because of adverse events.

COMMENT

Topical retinoids are considered core of topical therapy in acne as they resolve the precursor lesions of inflammatory acne, the microcomedones. Topical retinoids also block several important inflammatory pathways that are activated in acne: toll-like receptors, leukocyte migration, and the activator protein 1 (AP-1) pathway. They are also used for maintenance therapy. In addition to affecting primary acne lesions, topical retinoids have also been shown to act on secondary lesions including scarring and pigmentation because of actions in the dermis. In pigmentary problems, topical retinoids lighten hyperpigmented lesions by inhibiting melanosome transfer to keratinocytes and reducing epidermal pigmentation by accelerating epidermal turnover. In this study, authors have evaluated the efficacy and safety of lotion preparation of tretinoin. A total of 1,640 patients aged 9–58 years were included in the study. It was a 12-week, double-blind, randomized, vehicle-controlled study. Tretinoin 0.05% lotion demonstrated statistically significant superiority to vehicle in reducing inflammatory and noninflammatory lesion counts at week 12 and improving acne severity. About 50% change in the inflammatory and noninflammatory lesions was seen by week 12. Tretinoin 0.05% lotion was very well tolerated with no substantive differences in cutaneous tolerability among treatment groups. No patients discontinued the treatment because of adverse events.

> **Key Message**
>
> - Tretinoin 0.05% lotion provides statistically significant greater efficacy than vehicle with a highly favorable safety and tolerability profile in moderate-to-severe acne patients.

ARTICLE 3

Once-daily Oral Sarecycline 1.5 mg/kg/day is Effective for Moderate-to-severe Acne Vulgaris: Results from Two Identically Designed, Phase 3, Randomized, Double-blind Clinical Trials

Moore A, Green LJ, Bruce S, et al. Once-Daily Oral Sarecycline 1.5 mg/kg/day Is Effective for Moderate to Severe Acne Vulgaris: Results from Two Identically Designed, Phase 3, Randomized, Double-Blind Clinical Trials.
J Drugs Dermatol. 2018;17(9):987-96.

Abstract

Tetracyclines are the most commonly used antibiotics in acne because of their antibiotic and anti-inflammatory profile. The objective of this study was to evaluate the efficacy and safety of once-daily sarecycline in moderate-to-severe acne. Sarecycline is the first narrow-spectrum tetracycline antibiotic used in acne. The patients were treated with sarecycline 1.5 mg/kg for 12 weeks. The reduction in the inflammatory lesions was noted at 3 weeks and noninflammatory lesions were noted at 6 weeks. The side effects like nausea, headache, and photosensitivity occurred in less than 2% and were considered as not treatment related. Sarecycline is safe and effective in moderate-to-severe acne, with minimal side effects.

COMMENT

Isotretinoin and tetracycline groups of antibiotics are the commonly used medications in moderate-to-severe acne. Tetracyclines have been widely used for the treatment of moderate-to-severe acne due to their ability to suppress the growth of *Cutibacterium acnes*—an anaerobic organism associated with acne lesions—and their ability to exert anti-inflammatory effects. Common side effects of tetracyclines are nausea, diarrhea, loss of appetite, giddiness, headache and fatigue. Though minocycline is effective, its side effects, especially pigmentation of the skin, limit its extensive use in acne. In this study, the efficacy and safety of sarecycline was evaluated in moderate-to-severe acne.

Sarecycline is the first narrow-spectrum tetracycline class antibiotic developed for acne treatment. In addition to exhibiting activity against important skin/soft tissue pathogens, sarecycline exhibits targeted antibacterial activity against clinical isolates of *Cutibacterium acnes*. In previous study, it was shown that sarecycline was 16- to 32-fold less active than broad-spectrum tetracyclines—such as minocycline and doxycycline—against aerobic gram-negative bacilli associated with the normal human intestinal microbiome. Sarecycline was also 4- to 8-fold less active than doxycycline against representative anaerobic bacteria that also comprise the normal human intestinal microbiome.

Sarecycline was used in dose of 1.5 mg/kg and tested against a placebo in patients with moderate-to-severe acne lesions. Onset in the reduction of inflammatory lesions was noticed as early as 3 weeks, and onset of efficacy for absolute reduction of noninflammatory lesion count occurred at week 6 and week 9. About 4% of patients complained of nausea and 2% complained of headache and vomiting. Most of these side effects were considered as not treatment related. Vestibular (dizziness, tinnitus and vertigo) and phototoxic (sunburn and photosensitivity) occurred in less than 1%.

Key Message

- The narrow-spectrum antibiotic, sarecycline was safe, well tolerated, and effective for moderate-to-severe acne, with low rates of side effects common with tetracycline antibiotics.

ARTICLE 4

The Efficacy and Safety of Azelaic Acid 15% Foam in the Treatment of Facial Acne Vulgaris

Hashim PW, Chen T, Harper JC, et al. The Efficacy and Safety of Azelaic Acid 15% Foam in the Treatment of Facial Acne Vulgaris.
J Drugs Dermatol. 2018;17(6):641-5.

Abstract

Azelaic acid has anti-inflammatory, antioxidative, anticomedogenic, and antimicrobial effects. Azelaic acid 20% cream has been approved for the treatment of acne vulgaris, and azelaic acid 15% foam has been approved for rosacea. Given the favorable tolerability profile of foam preparations, it is reasonable to assume that azelaic acid 15% foam could serve as a viable treatment option for facial acne. The objective of this study was to examine the efficacy and safety of azelaic acid 15% foam in the treatment of moderate-to-severe facial acne. The authors concluded that all the subjects experienced reductions in lesion count by week 16 and was well tolerated by patients.

COMMENT

The etiopathogenesis of acne is multifactorial, as a result of which no single agent is going to be very effective in acne. Azelaic acid is a naturally occurring dicarboxylic acid analog. It is found in some grains and also in our body in small amounts. It has antimicrobial as well as keratinization-normalizing function. About 20% azelaic acid cream has been used in acne. About 15% foam preparation is approved for use in rosacea. As the foam preparation has a better patient tolerability profile, the authors have studied the efficacy and safety of 15% foam preparation of azelaic acid in mild-to-moderate acne. The study duration was 6 weeks. There was significant reduction in the number of both inflammatory and noninflammatory lesions. The usual side effects of cream like erythema, itching, burning, and peeling of skin were not noticed with this foam preparation.

Key Message

- Azelaic acid 15% foam is effective and safe in the treatment of facial acne vulgaris.

ARTICLE 5

Frequency of Treatment Switching for Spironolactone Compared to Oral Tetracycline-class Antibiotics for Women with Acne: A Retrospective Cohort Study 2010–2016

Barbieri JS, Choi JK, Mitra N, et al. Frequency of Treatment Switching for Spironolactone Compared to Oral Tetracycline-Class Antibiotics for Women With Acne: A Retrospective Cohort Study 2010-2016.
J Drugs Dermatol. 2018;17(6):632-8.

Abstract

Acne is a chronic disorder. Moderate-to-severe acne requires long-term therapy. Oral antibiotics are commonly prescribed in acne. The long-term use of these antibiotics may result in resistance and complications like pharyngitis. The objective of this study was to analyze the frequency of treatment switching for spironolactone as compared to tetracycline. A retrospective analysis of the frequency of switching to different systemic agents in 1st year of acne therapy was done. It was reported that among women who were started on spironolactone, 14.4% were prescribed another systemic agent within 1 year as compared to 13.4% of patients who were prescribed tetracycline.

Results: As the rate of switching between spironolactone and systemic antibiotics are similar, it may be concluded that the clinical effectiveness is also similar. Spironolactone may be considered as an alternative to tetracycline.

COMMENT

Acne is a common chronic disorder and therapy in acne is usually prolonged. Systemic therapy for moderate-to-severe acne consists of oral isotretinoin and tetracycline group of antibiotics. Antibiotics when prescribed over a long period may be associated with side effects like resistance, pharyngitis. Spironolactone is an androgen receptor antagonist. As androgens have a role in pathogenesis of acne by increasing sebum production, spironolactone has been accepted as a therapy in acne. Spironolactone may be considered as a safe alternative to long-term use of antibiotics. Spironolactone is quite safe in women and its side effects like hyperkalemia or breast cancer have not been supported by evidence. A retrospective analysis was conducted to analyze the frequency of switching of different systemic agents within the 1st year of therapy. Patients who were prescribed spironolactone or tetracycline antibiotics were included in the study. It was reported that among women who were started on spironolactone, 14.4% were prescribed another systemic agent within 1 year as compared to 13.4% of patients who were prescribed tetracycline. Based on the observation of similar switching between the two groups, spironolactone may have similar clinical effectiveness to that of oral tetracycline-class antibiotics.

Spironolactone cannot replace tetracycline group of antibiotics in acne. It cannot be used in males due to the side effect like gynecomastia. Common side effects of long-term use of spironolactone during treatment for acne include irregular menstruation, urinary frequency, dizziness, headaches, nausea, vomiting, breast tenderness, and breast enlargement. So till further studies are available on large scale, tetracyclines continue to be used more commonly in acne.

Key Message

- As the rate of switching between spironolactone and systemic antibiotics are similar, it may be concluded that the clinical effectiveness is also similar. Spironolactone may be considered as an alternative to tetracycline.

ARTICLE 6

Clinical Experience with Once-daily Dapsone Gel, 7.5% Monotherapy in Patients with Acne Vulgaris

Stockton TC, Tanghetti EA, Lain E, et al. Clinical Experience with Once-Daily Dapsone Gel, 7.5% Monotherapy in Patients with Acne Vulgaris.
J Drugs Dermatol. 2018;17(6):602-8.

Abstract

Topical dapsone 7.5% gel is approved for acne in patients above 12 years of age. The objective of this study was to study the efficacy of dapsone 7.5% gel as monotherapy for acne. Patients were treated for 12 weeks and assessed for efficacy and side effects. Dapsone monotherapy was efficacious in treating moderate acne without any severe adverse events.

COMMENT

Management of acne is based on the clinical severity. Mild-to-moderate acne is treated with topical therapy and severe acne with systemic therapy. In topical therapy, topical retinoids and benzoyl peroxide are used as first-line therapy, usually. Topical antibiotics are not prescribed as sole medications due to the risk of development of resistance. Topical antibiotics are usually combined with topical tretinoin or benzoyl peroxide.

In this study, the patients were treated with dapsone 7.5% gel as monotherapy. Eight patients were enrolled in the study and the duration of study was 12 weeks. Patients were evaluated at baseline and after 12 weeks. Result was assessed based on clinical photographs, dermatologist assessment, and patient comments. All patients tolerated the topical dapsone gel; there were no reported side effects. Significant improvement was seen in all patients who were prescribed acne monotherapy.

Key Message
- As dapsone is an antibiotic, there is a risk of development of resistance with monotherapy of dapsone.

ARTICLE 7

An Acne Survey from the World's Largest Annual Gathering of Twins

Suggs A, Loesch M, Ezaldein H, et al. An Acne Survey from the World's Largest Annual Gathering of Twins. *J Drugs Dermatol. 2018;17(4):380-2.*

Abstract

In this study, identical twins were studied to qualitatively separate genetic factors from environmental factors. The objective of this study was to identify environmental factors that influence severity of acne. The study reported that acne was associated with polycystic ovarian syndrome, anxiety and asthma. Twins with acne had a higher body mass index (BMI) and exercised less. Those with more severe acne reported aggravation of acne with cosmetic product use.

COMMENT

Studies done on identical twins help us to distinguish between genetic and environmental factors for acne. From our clinical experience, we know that acne runs in families, especially severe acne and scarring. A study, published in 2002 by Bativelle et al. showed that 81% of variance of the disease was attributable to additive genetic effects. Apolipoprotein A1 serum levels were found to be lower in twins with acne. Here, the authors have surveyed 139 identical and fraternal twins at the Annual Twins Day Festival in Twinsburg, Ohio on August 6-7, 2016. They measured the incidence of acne, severity and triggers. The concordance was found to be more with identical twins. Acne was found to be associated with polycystic ovarian syndrome, anxiety and asthma. It was also found that twins with acne exercised less frequently and had higher BMI.

Key Message
- This twin study further supports that there may be a genetic phenotypic link, though social and environmental factors may also have an influence in the disease process.

ARTICLE 8

Efficacy and Safety of Adapalene 0.3%/Benzoyl Peroxide 2.5% Gel plus Oral Doxycycline in Subjects with Severe Inflammatory Acne who are Candidates for Oral Isotretinoin

Del Rosso JQ, Stein Gold L, Johnson SM, et al. Efficacy and Safety of Adapalene 0.3%/Benzoyl Peroxide 2.5% Gel Plus Oral Doxycycline in Subjects with Severe Inflammatory Acne who are Candidates for Oral Isotretinoin. *J Drugs Dermatol.* 2018;17(3):264-273.

Abstract

Mild-to-moderate acne is managed with topical retinoid and benzoyl peroxide. In systemic therapy for acne, the first-line options are isotretinoin and tetracycline group of antibiotic. In this study, the efficacy of daily regimen of 0.3% adapalene and 2.5% benzoyl peroxide (0.3% A/BPO) gel and oral doxycycline 100 mg twice daily in severe (non-nodulocystic, nonconglobate) inflammatory acne was evaluated. The results were satisfactory with significant improvement in acne scores.

COMMENT

Isotretinoin is considered as the gold standard in grade 4 acne vulgaris and severe acne. Commonly used topical therapies are benzoyl peroxide and topical retinoids. Among the tetracycline group of antibiotics, doxycycline is commonly used for acne. Treatment for moderate-to-severe acne is usually combination of topical and systemic therapies. In this study, done for 12 weeks, patients were treated with doxycycline, adapalene/benzoyl peroxide combination. Endpoint for efficacy was reduction in inflammatory lesions. Significant reduction in acne inflammatory lesions was noted at the end of 12 weeks, and also most patients were satisfied with the treatment. Only 19% of patients were still considered to have severe acne at the end of the study.

Key Message

- Combination of adapalene, benzoyl peroxide, and doxycycline is a safe and effective alternative in treatment of severe acne vulgaris. It can also be used in patients in whom isotretinoin is contraindicated.

ARTICLE 9

Efficacy, Safety and Tolerability of Topical Dapsone Gel, 7.5% for Treatment of Acne Vulgaris by Fitzpatrick Skin Phototype

Taylor SC, Cook-Bolden FE, McMichael A, et al. Efficacy, Safety, and Tolerability of Topical Dapsone Gel, 7.5% for Treatment of Acne Vulgaris by Fitzpatrick Skin Phototype.
J Drugs Dermatol. 2018;17(2):160-7.

Abstract

Acne vulgaris in patients with skin of color has a higher sequel-like scarring and hyperpigmentation compared to their counterparts with light skin. In this study, the difference in tolerability and response to dapsone 7.5% was evaluated depending on the Fitzpatrick skin phototype. There was no difference in side effect profile or efficacy of dapsone among various skin phototypes.

COMMENT

Acne vulgaris is universal irrespective of skin types. The prevalence of acne is about 80% during adolescence. The unfortunate sequela of acne scarring is higher in skin of color. Dapsone 5% is routinely used in the management of acne. Dapsone is a sulfone antibiotic and also has anti-inflammatory action. Because of this dual action, it is suitable for acne management. Systemic dapsone on long-term use has potential for side effects. Topical dapsone allows clinically effective doses of dapsone to be administered topically with minimal systemic absorption.

In this study, the differences in response and tolerability to dapsone gel 7.5% were compared among the various skin color types. In this double-blind, randomized, vehicle-controlled study, patients were asked to apply either 7.5% dapsone gel or vehicle daily for 12 weeks. A total of 2,216 patients with skin phototypes I–III and 2,111 with phototypes IV–VI were included and evaluated. Dapsone significantly improved the severity of acne in both the groups. Considerable reduction was noted in the inflammatory and comedonal lesions. No side effects were reported by any of the patients.

Key Message
- Once-daily dapsone gel, 7.5% was effective, safe, and well tolerated in patients with all skin phototypes who were treated for moderate acne.

ARTICLE 10

Clinical Significance of Neutrophil Gelatinase-associated Lipocalin and Galectin-7 in Tape-stripped Stratum Corneum of Acne Vulgaris

Watanabe K, Yoshino T, Takahashi M, et al. Clinical significance of neutrophil gelatinase-associated lipocalin and galectin-7 in tape-stripped stratum corneum of acne vulgaris.
J Dermatol. 2018;45(5):618-21.

Abstract

In this study, the authors have studied the levels of neutrophil gelatinase-associated lipocalin (NGAL) levels and galectin-7 levels in patients with acne before and after therapy. It was done to see the utility of the above molecules as biomarkers for acne severity. The study showed a significant decrease in the NGAL levels with therapy on cheek skin.

COMMENT

Acne is a common disorder of adolescence with significant psychological morbidity in severe cases. This study was conducted to evaluate the role of neutrophil gelatinase-associated lipocalin (NGAL) as a biomarker for the severity of acne. NGAL was initially isolated from neutrophils and is expressed in the infundibulum of hair follicle; it reaches the skin surface through the sebum flowing via the follicular ducts. Galectin-7 is expressed during epidermal differentiation and plays a role in maintaining epidermal homeostasis. Previous studies have shown that epidermal disruption or disturbance in barrier function is associated with increased galectin levels. Tape stripping of stratum corneum was done in study subjects and the sample evaluated for NGAL and galectin-7. The study showed increase in NGAL level of cheek samples in patients with acne and reduction in the levels with treatment. As, with treatment, inflammation reduces, NGAL level may be utilized as an inflammatory biomarker for acne to check the severity. However, its relevance in clinical practice is yet to be established. Also to be noted is that the reduction after treatment was noted only in cheek samples and not the stratum corneum samples from the forehead.

Key Message
- Neutrophil gelatinase-associated lipocalin can be used as a biomarker for severity of acne.

ARTICLE 11

Risk of Depression among Patients with Acne: A Population-based Cohort Study using The Health Improvement Network (THIN) Database

Vallerand I, Lewinson R, Parsons L, et al. Risk of depression among patients with acne: A population-based cohort study using The Health Improvement Network (THIN) database.
J Am Acad Dermatol. 2018;79(3):AB247.

Abstract

Acne is a common chronic skin disorder, which sometimes causes severe psychological morbidity. The decreased self-esteem due to acne sometimes leads to major depressive disorder. This study was conducted to evaluate the risk of depression among acne patients. Acne was found to be associated with depression, especially in patients who sought medical advice. The depressive symptoms decreased over 5 years.

COMMENT

Acne is a common skin disorder usually seen in adolescents. During adolescence, the prevalence of acne is higher in boys. However, the anxiety and stress associated with acne are more common among girls. It was shown earlier that adolescent girls were more susceptible to the negative psychological effects of acne. Twice as many girls as boys were reported to have depression.

There are many studies where it has been reported that there is increased prevalence of depression among acne patients as compared to the general population. Depression was found to be two to three times more in patients with acne, and these symptoms reduce considerably after effective treatment. Aggressive treatment of acne is necessary to prevent anxiety and also reduces complications like scarring, which will further cause long time psychological distress. The relationship between severity of acne and depressive symptoms is not consistent with various studies.

Key Message

- Acne causes reduced self-esteem and is associated with major depressive disorder in few. While treating patients, physicians should be aware of these symptoms, as few may need referral to mental health services.

ARTICLE 12

Acne Development in Male Androgenetic Alopecia

Rajan A, Grotts J, Goh C. Acne development in male androgenetic alopecia.
Clin Exp Dermatol. 2019;44(3):e39-e40.

Abstract

Acne and androgenetic alopecia (AGA) have been linked in females through hyperandrogenism conditions like polycystic ovarian syndrome (PCOS). A retrospective study was conducted to see the association of acne and AGA in male patients. The study concluded that there is increased association of acne with AGA, especially adult acne.

COMMENT

Early androgenetic alopecia (AGA) in men is reported to be the phenotypic equivalent of polycystic ovarian syndrome (PCOS) in women. PCOS carries an increased risk of developing obesity, metabolic syndrome, and cardiovascular diseases. Metabolic studies of patients with early AGA have been found to be similar to that of PCOS. In this retrospective study, association of acne in patients with AGA was evaluated against healthy controls who did not have AGA. In this study, a significant association between acne and AGA was noted, especially adult acne. However, hair loss induced due to isotretinoin therapy for acne could not be evaluated. This association can be explained by the role of androgens in both these conditions. Various studies of hormonal profiles of patients with AGA have supported that AGA might be phenotypic equivalent of PCOS. Thus, AGA might be considered as part of systemic condition of hyperandrogenism, in which there is higher incidence of complications from diabetes, coronary artery disease, and insulin resistance.

Key Message

- The increased association of adult acne in AGA may be because both are androgen-induced conditions.

ARTICLE 13

Effects of Isotretinoin Treatment on Affective and Cognitive Functions in Adolescent Acne Vulgaris Patients

Maden A, Kocyigit P. Effects of isotretinoin treatment on affective and cognitive functions in adolescent acne vulgaris patients.
J Am Acad Dermatol. 2018;79(3):AB118.

Abstract

The causal relationship between isotretinoin and depression is not established. This study was conducted to study if isotretinoin has any role in affective and cognitive functions in adolescents. The study concluded that none of the patients fulfilled clinical depression criteria with isotretinoin.

COMMENT

The risk of depression with isotretinoin has been a matter of debate for a long time. The causal relationship between isotretinoin and depression is not established. However, it seems to have a positive psychological impact in majority of severe acne patients due to its efficacy. Majority of other studies, which were conducted to evaluate the association of isotretinoin and depression, have shown that there is actual improvement in symptoms. Oral isotretinoin significantly suppressed cell division in the hippocampus and severely disrupted the learning capacity of mice in a study by Crandall et al. As hippocampus and prefrontal cortex are involved in mood regulation and cognitive function, this study was conducted to study the impact of isotretinoin on cognitive functions. Neuropsychological test battery and psychometric tests were used to assess cognitive functions. The tests were performed before starting therapy and 3 months after the therapy. None of the patients fulfilled clinical depression criteria and in fact consistent with other studies there was improvement in attention and memory in these patients.

Key Message
- *Isotretinoin does not cause significant depression of cognitive functions.*

ARTICLE 14

Analysis of Gut Microbiome in Patients with Acne Vulgaris

Hitosugi N. Analysis of Gut Microbiome in Patients with Acne Vulgaris.
J Am Acad Dermatol. 2018;79(3):AB42.

Abstract

Gut microbiome components have been implicated in various diseases. In this study, authors have compared gut microbiome of patients with acne vulgaris with that of controls and found that firmicutes was significantly increased in acne patients.

COMMENT

The human intestine hosts diverse bacterial species that reside mostly in the lower gut maintaining a symbiosis with the human habitat. Salem et al. published gut microbiome as a major regulator of skin gut axis. The complex connection between acne and gastrointestinal (GI) dysfunction may also be mediated by the brain, an idea first postulated by Stokes in 1930. Gut microbiota influence the pathophysiology of acne via cross-talk between intestinal commensal bacteria and the mTOR pathway as proposed by Noureldein et al. In this study, authors have compared the gut microbiota of patients with acne against those of control population. There is significant increase in firmicutes in patients with acne, resulting in a low ratio of bacteroides to firmicutes. Firmicutes decompose polysaccharides in the gut. No difference in actinobacteria and proteobacteria was noted. The clinical implication and causal association with acne is yet to be established.

Key Message

- *Firmicutes is increased in the gut of patients with acne vulgaris.*

ARTICLE 15

Isotretinoin Therapy: A Retrospective Cohort Analysis of Completion Rates and Factors Associated with Nonadherence

Kazemi T, Sachsman SM, Wilhalme HM, et al. Isotretinoin therapy: A retrospective cohort analysis of completion rates and factors associated with nonadherence.
J Am Acad Dermatol. 2018;79(3):571-3.

Abstract

Adherence to medications is the primary requirement for the therapy to be effective. The cumulative dose-dependent mechanism is important in maintaining remissions with isotretinoin. The authors have evaluated the factors associated with nonadherence and concluded that most common factor of nonadherence was failure to return for follow-ups. Commonly cited reason for discontinuation was mood changes, and iPLEDGE difficulties were the most common reason for failure to initiate treatment.

COMMENT

The primary cause for treatment failure in acne patients is nonadherence to treatment. Adherence to medication is necessary with isotretinoin, which has a cumulative dose-dependent mechanism in inducing emission. The authors did a retrospective review of 544 cases of isotretinoin prescriptions to check for nonadherence and the causes for that. Out of the 458 patients enrolled, 53.9% completed the therapy, 18.3% likely completed the therapy, 15.5% were lost to follow-up, 5.9% stopped due to physician orders, 4.2% self-discontinued, and 3.1% never started the therapy. Excluding the never started and physician-stopped group, adherence rate was 78.6% in this study. No significant difference in age and sex parameters was noticed between the adherent and nonadherent group. Among the lost to follow-up group, the number of men was significantly more. As the study was retrospective, the reasons for lost to follow-up could not be elucidated. The most common cause for not completing therapy was the loss to follow-up, i.e. missing the first follow-up appointment. Among the patients who discontinued medications on their own or advice of the physician, common reason cited was mood changes. Others reasons were being travel and unwillingness to stop alcohol. Most common reason cited for noninitiation of therapy was iPLEDGE difficulties.

Key Message

- Proper screening of patients and counseling about iPLEDGE before starting isotretinoin therapy will help patients adhere to therapy.

ARTICLE 16

Photodynamic Therapy for Acne Conglobata of the Buttocks: Effective Anti-inflammatory Treatment with Good Cosmetic Outcome

Borgia F, Vaccaro M, Giuffrida R, et al. Photodynamic therapy for acne conglobata of the buttocks: Effective antiinflammatory treatment with good cosmetic outcome.
Indian J Dermatol Venereol Leprol. 2018;84(5):617-9.

Abstract

Acne conglobata is a rare severe variant of acne, which is often difficult to treat and heals with scars. Here, authors reported the use of photodynamic therapy (PDT) in a young male patient of acne conglobata with satisfying results.

COMMENT

Acne conglobata is a rare severe form of acne affecting deep tissues causing swelling, purulent discharge, pain, and healing with disfiguring scars. These lesions are often resistant to treatment causing significant psychological morbidity in patients. Treatment options include isotretinoin and tetracycline group of antibiotics.

The authors have treated a 16-year-old male with lesions of acne conglobata limited to gluteal area with photodynamic therapy (PDT). PDT was considered when the patient's lesions did not improve with minocycline and isotretinoin. Sessions were done every 2 weeks for 3 months. Remarkable improvement was seen at the end of 3 months and the patient was in remission after 6 months of follow-up. Intense pain and inflammation were noticed after the first two sessions. No other side effects were noted, and the scarring was also minimal.

Photodynamic therapy has anti-inflammatory as well as antibacterial effects. During PDT, singlet oxygen species are released, which trigger apoptosis and cell necrosis. The greater absorption of aminolevulinic acid together with higher production of protoporphyrin IX in hair follicles compared to other tissues seems to be the mechanism of action in inflammatory diseases of the pilosebaceous unit such as chronic folliculitis, hidradenitis suppurativa, and probably in acne conglobata. The use of PDT in the early lesions may help in faster resolution of lesions and prevent disfiguring scars.

Key Message

- The good safety profile and absence of severe side effects make PDT a good option in the management of acne conglobata.

ARTICLE 17

Acneiform Eruptions: An Unusual Dermatological Side Effect of Ribavirin

Gupta M, Aggarwal M, Bhari N. Acneiform eruptions: An unusual dermatological side effect of ribavirin. *Dermatol Ther. 2018;31(5):e12679.*

Abstract

Acne vulgaris is a common skin disorder usually seen in adolescents. Drug-induced acne has been reported with systemic steroids, epidermal growth factor inhibitors, and danazol. Here, the authors have reported acneiform eruptions with ribavirin.

COMMENT

Acne vulgaris is a common disorder of adolescence with comedones, papules, pustules and nodules. Drug-induced acne has been reported with corticosteroid, epidermal growth factor receptor inhibitors, interferon-beta, granulocyte colony-stimulating factor, anti-tumor necrosis factor, sirolimus, tacrolimus, danazol and dantrolene. These lesions are monomorphic and widespread, involving face, chest, back and arms. Drug-induced acneiform eruptions regress considerably on stopping the medications.

The authors have reported a case of a 35-year-old man who presented with multiple papulonodular lesions on the face, neck, arms, and trunk 2 weeks after taking medications for chronic hepatitis C. Patient was treated with oral sofosbuvir 400 mg, daclatasvir 60 mg, and ribavirin 1,000 mg. He had acne in adolescents, with acne scars on bilateral cheeks.

On discontinuation of ribavirin, the lesions improved over the next 2 weeks. Sofosbuvir and daclatasvir were continued.

Ribavirin is a commonly used drug in chronic hepatitis C. Hepatitis C is associated with type II mixed cryoglobulinemia, lichen planus, porphyria cutanea tarda, chronic pruritus, necrolytic acral erythema, and several immune-mediated inflammatory skin conditions, such as psoriasis, chronic urticaria and vitiligo. The known cutaneous side effects of ribavirin are alopecia, skin rash, xeroderma, dermatitis, diaphoresis, erythema multiforme, erythroderma, vesiculobullous reaction, Stevens–Johnson syndrome, and toxic epidermal necrolysis.

Key Message
- Acneiform eruptions as a possible side effect of ribavirin should be kept in mind along with other dermatological side effects.

ARTICLE 18

Topical Dapsone Gel is a New Treatment Option for Acne Agminata

Ferguson L, Fearfield L. Topical dapsone gel is a new treatment option for acne agminata.
Clin Exp Dermatol. 2019;44(4):453-5.

Abstract

Acne agminata is characterized by papular lesions predominantly on centrofacial areas of the face. The exact etiology is unknown and there is no specific defined treatment. Systemic steroids, isotretinoin, doxycycline, and dapsone are commonly used medications. Here, the authors report successful management of acne agminata with topical dapsone for over a year, without any significant adverse effects.

COMMENT

Acne agminata, also known as lupus miliaris disseminatus faciei or facial idiopathic granulomas with regressive evolution (FIGURE), is a rare granulomatous condition of unknown etiology commonly affecting the centrofacial area. Histopathology shows tuberculoid granulomas in the mid dermis, sometimes with variants. There is lack of evidence of a single effective therapy in acne agminata. Commonly used medications are systemic steroids, isotretinoin, doxycycline, clofazimine, and oral dapsone.

The authors, have reported successful treatment of 31-year-old patient of acne agminata with topical dapsone 5%. This patient was treated with prednisolone for 1 month, lymecycline for 3 months, and 2 courses of isotretinoin for 6 months each without significant improvement. Patient was prescribed topical dapsone 5% gel twice daily, significant improvement with reduced size of papules was seen at 3 months. When dapsone was stopped at 6 months, patient had a flare-up of lesions, for which the gel was continued. Treatment was stopped at 11 months without any further recurrence. There were no cutaneous side effects and blood investigations before and after treatment were also normal. Topical dapsone has a good long- and short-term safety data. There is a risk of methemoglobinemia with topical dapsone also, so it should be avoided in individuals with glucose-6-phosphate dehydrogenase (G6PD) deficiency. Topical dapsone can also be used as an adjunct to topical steroids or isotretinoin in acne agminata.

Key Messages
- Topical dapsone gel can be used for treatment of acne agminata, it has a good safety profile
- As there is risk of methemoglobinemia with topical dapsone also, it should be avoided in individuals with G6PD deficiency.

ARTICLE 19

The Effect of Continuous High versus Low Dose Oral Isotretinoin Regimens on Dermcidin Expression in Patients with Moderate-to-severe Acne Vulgaris

El Aziz Ragab MA, Omar SS, Collier A, et al. The effect of continuous high versus low dose oral isotretinoin regimens on dermcidin expression in patients with moderate to severe acne vulgaris.
Dermatol Ther. 2018;31(6):e12715.

Abstract

Dermcidin is an antimicrobial peptide with a broad spectrum of activity against bacteria such as *Propionibacterium acnes* (*P. acnes*). Level of dermcidin is low in acne vulgaris. This study was conducted to evaluate the effects of continuous low dose and conventional doses of isotretinoin on dermcidin levels. Both regimens caused a significant increase in the levels of dermcidin compared to pretreatment values, and the relapse after 12 months was not statistically different among the two regimens.

COMMENT

Antimicrobial peptides play a role in acne vulgaris. Few act by reducing *P. acnes* and others may have proinflammatory effects. Dermcidin is a protein expressed in sweat glands and sebaceous glands with antibacterial and antifungal properties. Nakano et al. in 2015 had proposed that low levels of dermcidin in acne patients allow proliferation of *P. acnes* and promote inflammation. Dermcidin probably promotes the growth of regular flora, which reduces *P. acnes* colonization.

In this study, the authors have measured dermcidin levels in 30 patients of acne vulgaris from the skin biopsy samples using ELISA (enzyme-linked immunosorbent assay) technique. Biopsies were done at the beginning of the treatment and again at the end of 6 months. About 15 patients were prescribed low-dose isotretinoin, i.e. 20 mg/day, and 15 patients were prescribed the conventional dose of 0.5 mg/day. About 15 patients without acne vulgaris were considered as controls. Patients were followed up again at the end of 6 months for relapse.

Patients with acne had a lower level of dermcidin as compared to controls. On treatment, the dermcidin levels increased significantly in both the regimens, the clinical improvement was significantly related to increase in the dermcidin levels. Relapse was also significantly related to post-treatment dermcidin level. The two regimens of isotretinoin did not show any significant difference in change of dermcidin levels.

Isotretinoin is known to increase the expression of psoriasin and lipocalin-2 in acne patients. This study proves that isotretinoin-induced dermcidin upregulation may also contribute in its anti-acne effects.

Key Messages

- Low dose and conventional doses of isotretinoin did not show significant differences in clinical improvement in moderate acne
- Isotretinoin may exert its anti-acne effect by upregulation of dermcidin, which has anti-P. acnes properties.

ARTICLE 20

Transgender Adolescents and Acne: A Case Series

Campos-Muñoz L, López-De Lara D, Rodríguez-Rojo ML, et al. Transgender adolescents and acne: A case series. *Pediatr Dermatol. 2018;35(3):e155-8.*

Abstract

Female-to-male transgender adolescents are treated with testosterone. Acne is a foreseeable side effect in them. The authors have outlined the difficulties in treating transgender adolescents for acne, the drug interactions, concerns of hepatotoxicity with medications, and psychological aspects.

COMMENT

Transgenderism is incongruence between a person's somatic sex and the sex with which a person identifies emotionally and psychologically, lasting for more than 6 months. In female-to-male transgenders, testosterone is prescribed for masculinizing effects. This is associated with acne and androgenetic alopecia as cutaneous side effects. As acne is a known side effect, treatment has to be provided even in mild cases, as the psychological stress from acne can be huge.

The authors treated five transgender patients of acne, two with isotretinoin 20 mg/day and remaining with doxycycline. Liver function tests were monitored every 8 weeks and were normal. Four of these patients had acne even before starting testosterone therapy, but in all of them, acne aggravated after testosterone. Antiandrogens and oral contraceptives cannot be prescribed in these cases for acne, as it would conflict with the masculinizing effects of testosterone.

The possibility of intrahepatic cholestasis is described with testosterone. Similarly, a greater likelihood of hepatotoxicity is described with tetracyclines and isotretinoin. As female-to-male transgender individuals are treated exclusively with testosterone, frequent monitoring of liver function tests is recommended when the acne is treated with isotretinoin or tetracyclines.

In patients with natal female genitalia, there is a risk of conception. Due to testosterone-induced amenorrhea, patients believe that the chances of pregnancy are null. However, pregnancy in female-to-male transgenders who were on testosterone has been described in literature. As isotretinoin is teratogenic, patients should be advised against pregnancy. Incidence of depression and suicidal tendencies is higher in transgenders compared to cisgenders. Appearance of severe acne might worsen underlying depression in them.

Key Messages

- Special considerations should be given when treating acne in transgender individuals; even mild acne should be treated
- Antiandrogens and oral contraceptives should not be prescribed in female-to-male transgender cases.

ARTICLE 21

Chemical Peels in the Treatment of Acne: Patient Selection and Perspectives

Castillo DE, Keri JE. Chemical peels in the treatment of acne: patient selection and perspectives. *Clin Cosmet Investig Dermatol.* 2018;11:365-72.

Abstract

This review article gives information regarding the most important factors to be considered while selecting a patient for a chemical peel, how to choose the peeling agent with respect to its safety and efficacy. This article also highlights about mechanism of action of different peeling agents along with their efficacy and safety in different races. Most of the peels are safe in Fitzpatrick skin type I–III. Deep peels to be avoided in darker skin types due to risk of hyperpigmentation and scarring. Proper selection of patient, peeling agent, preprocedure preparation of the skin along with appropriate postprocedure care minimizes the risk of complications.

COMMENT

Acne being the disease of adolescent has significant psychological impact. Among the various treatment modalities, chemical peels are one of the frequently performed cosmetic procedures as an adjuvant or monotherapy. The various peeling agents used in acne include salicylic acid (SA) (5–30%), which is sebostatic, bactericidal, and promotes shedding of epidermal cells; glycolic acid (GA) (20–70%); lactic acid (LA); mandelic acid (MA), which acts by decreasing corneocytes adhesion and exfoliation; trichloroacetic acid (TCA), which causes denaturation of epidermal and dermal proteins, destruction of dermal collagen, and coagulative necrosis of epidermal cells resulting in collagen and elastin remodulation; and kojic acid (KA), a copper-chelating agent, decreases tyrosinase activity acting as skin lightener. Apart from these, Jessner's solution (JS), a combination of 14% SA, 14% resorcinol, and 14% LA in 95% ethanol, is another commonly used peel in acne with individual agents with above described action and resorcinol causing disruption of the hydrogen bonds of keratin, disruption of cell membranes, and bactericidal agent. Phenol peels are very effective agents but they are less frequently used due to systemic toxic effects.

In Caucasians having a Fitzpatrick skin type I–III, various studies demonstrate safety of SA (20%) peel, GA (30%) peels, TCA (20%) peel in mild-to-moderate acne with very low risk of postinflammatory hyperpigmentation or scarring. In dark-skinned individuals (Fitzpatrick skin type IV–VI), patients are at greater risk of postinflammatory hypo- or hyperpigmentation and scarring. Though superficial peeling agents are safe, some experienced authors use medium-depth peels with good results. However, deep peels should be avoided due to the risk of hyperpigmentation and scarring. Studies demonstrate that both SA and GA peels are safe in these patients but should be used with precaution to avoid complications. In Asians with Fitzpatrick skin type III–V puts them at risk of post-peel complications. SA 20%, variable concentrations of GA peel (35%, 40% and 50%), and JS peels are safe and effective in Asians. TCA peel is associated with a greater risk of complications and should be avoided or used with caution. Not much studies are reported in Hispanic/Latinos with skin type Fitzpatrick skin type III–VI. Psychologically disturbed patients, patients with poor doctor–patient relationship, unrealistic expectations, infections, history of radiotherapy, hypertrophic or keloid scars, and immunosuppression, are not the ideal candidates for peel.

Complications that are common a few days or weeks following the procedure for every type of agent include swelling, erythema, pain and burning, pruritus, ecchymoses, blistering or infection, milia and telangiectasia. These can be minimized with preprocedure application of priming agents like topical retinoids and sunscreens for 6 weeks before the procedure and to be stopped 48 hours and 2–3 weeks prior to procedure in light- and dark-skinned individuals, respectively. It should be followed by strict photoprotection. Antiviral drugs should be added to prevent herpes reactivation. Post-peel pigmentation responds well to depigmenting agents like hydroquinone. Apart from local complications, SA and phenol peels, when used in large quantity, can result in systemic complications. In pregnancy, though safety is not established, GA and LA peels are considered safe due to poor dermal penetration, SA peel should be limited to small areas and TCA peels to be avoided in pregnancy.

Key Messages

- Superficial to medium-depth chemical peels are useful adjuvant therapies in acne vulgaris
- Choosing the type of agents depends on patient skin type and associated comorbidities
- Chemical peels are safe in light-colored skin. Deep peels should be avoided in darker skin types.

ARTICLE 22

A Novel Cognitive Stress Management Technique for Acne Vulgaris: A Short Report of a Pilot Experimental Study

Chatzikonstantinou F, Miskedaki A, Antoniou C, et al. A novel cognitive stress management technique for acne vulgaris: a short report of a pilot experimental study.
Int J Dermatol. 2019;58(2):218-20.

Abstract

This article analyzes effectiveness of a novel method, dubbed Pythagorean Self-Awareness Intervention (PSAI) in acne vulgaris (AV). This two-armed 1:1 randomized nonblind experimental study showed that PSAI is a feasible and possibly effective stress management method for AV.

COMMENT

Acne is a common skin disorder affecting the pilosebaceous unit and causing significant psychological morbidity among patients. One of the proposed mechanisms of pathogenesis is increased sebum production. Stress being a major regulator of the endocrine signaling influences sebum production both directly via the production of adrenal androgens, which are secreted simultaneously with cortisol and indirectly due to the influence of cortisol and central mediators of stress on the hypothalamic–pituitary–gonadal axis. In this study, the authors assessed the efficacy of cognitive-based stress management intervention and dubbed Pythagorean Self-Awareness Intervention (PSAI) to improve acne, acne-related quality of life, perceived stress and emotions.

Acne patients were randomized using an online generator into two groups one receiving intervention with PSAI for 8 weeks and the other group as control. PSAI comprised of eight weekly group sessions. During the first session, PSAI was introduced to the participants. This was followed by seven feedback and motivational group sessions. Patients practiced PSAI twice per day. Introspection and memory recall were two of the strongest tools used for achieving self-knowledge and self-mastery. At the end of the day, they were asked to recall every daily event in the exact time sequence that it happened. In the next step, each selected experience was critically appraised using certain fixed questions. Participants were advised to remain detached from any emotional burden and contemplate on the performed actions. Through positive (rejoice) and negative (reprimand) self-reinforcement, the individuals were asked to set certain specific goals for the next day after recapitulating the previous night's results, without repeating the procedure.

Patients were reassessed at the end of 8 weeks for acne stage. And the statistical analysis showed significant improvement in acne stage in intervention group. PSAI showed a large impact on stress and a moderate effect on negative affect. PSAI is an introspective method targeting to amend a dysfunctional situation, reduce stress and negative emotions. As compared to classical cognitive behavioral therapy, it is less time and money consuming and gives the opportunity to the individual to practice it at home, after a short period of appropriate training.

Key Messages

- Stress is a well-known aggravating factor in acne
- Along with the routine medical line of management, stress-relieving modalities offer significant control of the disease
- The PSAI is such an introspective method, which helps in alleviating stress thus achieving better control in acne patients.

ARTICLE 23

Evaluation of the Efficacy of Microneedle Fractional Radiofrequency in Turkish Patients with Atrophic Facial Acne Scars

Bulbul Baskan E, Akin Belli A. Evaluation of the efficacy of microneedle fractional radiofrequency in Turkish patients with atrophic facial acne scars.
J Cosmet Dermatol. 2018. [Epub ahead of print]

Abstract

This article analyzes safety and efficacy of microneedle fractional radiofrequency (MFR) in Turkish patients with atrophic facial acne scars. Patients with atrophic facial acne scars were subjected to MFR for average of three sittings at a gap of 4 weeks. Physicians' global assessment and patients' self-assessment scales done after 4 weeks after the last treatment session showed that a clinical improvement of >25% was seen in majority of patients and U-shaped atrophic acne scars responded better to the treatment than the other types, though not statistically significant.

COMMENT

Scarring is the permanent and distressing sequel of acne vulgaris. They can be hypertrophic or atrophic scars. Atrophic scars are subdivided into ice pick, rolling and box scars. Among the various treatment modalities, microneedle fractional radiofrequency (MFR) is the new emerging device with promising results. Effect mechanism of MFR involves microneedling, which is proven to enhance wound-healing response along with penetration of thermal energy into the reticular dermis without any superficial burns and thus induction of new collagen and elastin production and remodeling. This study aims to evaluate the efficacy and safety of MFR system in Turkish patients with atrophic facial acne scars.

In this retrospective study, clinical file of nine patients who underwent MFR were analyzed. Demographic profile and basic clinical information regarding severity, grading using Goodman and Barron's Global Qualitative Acne Scarring Grading System were recorded. After topical anesthesia and aseptic precautions, 25 insulated microneedles were performed with a median intensity of 70 W, a median needle depth of 3 mm, a median radiofrequency conduction time of 300 ms, and a median needle conduction time of 500 ms (range 450–550 ms). Postprocedure advice with sun protection, antibiotic and prophylactic antivirals were given. Average number of sittings undergone was three (one to five) at the interval of 4 weeks.

Accordingly, a clinical improvement of >25% was reported in seven patients (77.7%—physician) and eight patients (88.9%—patient). U-shaped atrophic acne scars achieved better clinical improvement than M type. Temporary pain, erythema, edema and crusting were the minimal and self-limiting side effect noted in the study. This article also highlights the outcome of various studies in which MFR is combined with subcision for optimum results. Literature analysis also shows that it is effective in the management of large pores. In conclusion, MFR system demonstrated a good efficacy and safety in Turkish patients with atrophic facial acne scars and had the advantage of quick return to daily life.

Key Messages

- Microneedle fractional radiofrequency is a combination of microneedling and radiofrequency both when applied enhance collegenogenesis
- As epidermis is not damaged, postprocedure complications are minimal
- Box scars respond well to MFR.

ARTICLE 24

Effect of Oral Isotretinoin on the Nucleocytoplasmic Distribution of FoxO1 and FoxO3 Proteins in Sebaceous Glands of Patients with Acne Vulgaris

Agamia NF, Hussein OM, Abdelmaksoud RE, et al. Effect of oral isotretinoin on the nucleo-cytoplasmic distribution of FoxO1 and FoxO3 proteins in sebaceous glands of patients with acne vulgaris.
Exp Dermatol. 2018;27(12):1344-51.

Abstract

Isotretinoin (13-cis-retinoic acid) is the most effective drug used in nodulocystic acne having sebum-suppressive action, which is brought about by sebocyte apoptosis. Isotretinoin-mediated apoptosis is thought to be due to increased nuclear activity of FoxO1 and other Fox transcription factors. One of the key proapoptotic proteins upregulated by isotretinoin in basal and suprabasal sebocytes is tumor necrosis factor-related apoptosis inducing ligand (TRAIL). Both FoxO1 and FoxO3 promote TRAIL expression. The aim of this study was to know if isotretinoin-induced TRAIL-mediated apoptosis in acne patients is associated with upregulated nuclear FoxO1 and FoxO3 proteins.

COMMENT

Though acne is considered as a disease of pilosebaceous unit, recently it was regarded as the metabolic syndrome promoted by attenuated overactivated mTORC1 signaling and Fox signaling of sebaceous glands. The aim of this study was to clarify whether isotretinoin-induced tumor necrosis factor-related apoptosis inducing ligand (TRAIL)-mediated apoptosis in acne patients may be associated with upregulated nuclear FoxO1 and FoxO3 proteins. Authors proposed that isotretinoin may preferentially increase nonphosphorylated Fox O transcription factors in the nucleus that may bring isotretinoin-mediated death signaling in targeted sebocytes. Phosphorylated and nonphosphorylated forms of FoxO1 and FoxO3 in sebaceous glands of patients with acne vulgaris were discriminated using commercial antibodies, which also determined the nucleocytoplasmic distribution of FoxO1 and FoxO3 before and 6 weeks after initiation of systemic isotretinoin treatment.

There was statistically significant difference in the cytoplasmic expression of non-p-FoxO1 antibody expression between the lesional and nonlesional specimen, but there was no statistically significant difference regarding nuclear expression of non-p-FoxO1 between the two specimens. There was a statistical significant difference between the lesional biopsies post-treatment with reduced non-p-FoxO1 in both nuclear and cytoplasmic compartment. The results were statistically significant in-between the nuclear expressions of p-FoxO1 antibody between the nonlesional and lesional specimens. No significant difference was noted between the lesional and nonlesional biopsies regarding cytoplasmic expression of p-FoxO1. There was no significant difference between lesional and nonlesional expression of the immunostain intensity, while there was a significant reduction in the stain intensity after treatment compared to the lesional and nonlesional biopsies. There was a significant statistical difference in the expression of p-FoxO1 immunostain in the lesional and after treatment biopsies between the nuclear and the cytoplasmic, respectively. The total amount of nuclear immunostain of FoxO1 had no significant difference between lesional, nonlesional and biopsies after isotretinoin treatment. The nucleocytoplasmic ratio of FoxO1 immunostain intensity showed that the stain was present much more in the cytoplasm. This ratio increased significantly ($p < 0.001$) after isotretinoin treatment. The difference in nuclear to cytoplasmic ratio of p-FoxO1 immunostain before treatment in the nonlesional biopsies in the acne lesions was not significant. This ratio was slightly increased after treatment and was not significant when compared to ratio before treatment in lesional biopsies, but was significant when compared to nonlesional biopsies. There was no statistical significant difference of non-p-FoxO3 antibody expression between the lesional and nonlesional specimen neither in the nuclear nor in the cytoplasmic compartment and after treatment as seen by image analysis and optical density for the immunohistochemical expression of FoxO3, cytoplasmic stain intensity decreased significantly with more nuclear concentration.

Total immunostain expression of FoxO3 analysis showed that there was no difference between lesional and nonlesional cytoplasmic expression of the immunostain intensity, while there was a significant decrease in the stain intensity after treatment. Neither was there any significant difference between lesional and nonlesional nor between lesional and after treatment biopsies for the nuclear intensity of total FoxO3 immunostain. However, there was a significant difference between nonlesional and after treatment biopsies. The nuclear to cytoplasmic ratio of FoxO3 immunostain intensity exhibited no significant difference in the ratio of non-p-FoxO3 immunostain before treatment in the nonlesional biopsies and in the acne lesions. However, the ratio reversed after treatment was indicating a nuclear concentration of non-p-FoxO3. There was no statistical significant difference regarding nuclear to cytoplasmic ratio of p-FoxO3 immunostain before treatment in the nonlesional biopsies and in the acne lesions, but this difference was significantly increased in biopsies after treatment, which indicates a moderate nuclear increase of p-FoxO3.

Key Messages
- Nuclear FoxO1 and FoxO3 are upregulated during isotretinoin treatment and potentially contribute to isotretinoin-mediated sebocyte apoptosis under in vivo conditions
- However, further research is required in this field.

ARTICLE 25

Adult-onset Acne: Prevalence, Impact and Management Challenges

Rocha MA, Bagatin E. Adult-onset acne: prevalence, impact, and management challenges. *Clin Cosmet Investig Dermatol. 2018;11:59-69.*

Abstract

This article reviews the epidemiological data regarding adult female acne. It analyzes the clinical features, prevalence of associated endocrine abnormalities, its impact and therapeutic options for adult female acne. Adult-onset acne is more common in females as compared to males. Only small percentage of these patients had associated endocrine abnormalities. When present, polycystic disease is the common condition. It significantly affects quality of life. Apart from conventional therapies, hormonal therapy is another effective option in these patients.

COMMENT

Though acne is described as disease of adolescents, very often it presents or persists after 25 years of age. Such incidence is more in females as compared to males. There are three types of adult acne. One which starts in adolescence and persists beyond the age of 25, second which starts at the age of 25, and the third being adolescent acne followed by acne free period to be followed by return of lesions in adult life. This adult acne, in contrast to adolescent acne, is distributed more on lower one-third of the face and side of the neck.

Various studies to know the association of endocrine abnormalities have shown that association is seen only in around one-third of the cases. In more than half of the patients, they failed to demonstrate any such association. However, it is suggested that, for the group of patients presenting with late-onset acne (at over 25 years of age), it is important to investigate the presence of endocrinological diseases than in patients with persistent acne.

The etiopathogenesis of acne is multifactorial. Immune-mediated and androgen-triggered acne, follicular hyperkeratinization, excess sebum production and innate immunity are known factors responsible for acne eruptions. In adult women, a positive correlation was observed between dihydrotestosterone (DHT), dehydroepiandrosterone sulfate (DHEAS) levels, and the inflammatory lesions severity, with blood levels of the insulin-like growth factor 1 (IGF-1). IGF-1 seems to mediate comedogenic factors such as androgens, growth hormone and glucocorticoids. Role of cosmetics remains controversial. Other factors that are considered as causative agent are stress and smoking.

From the endocrinological point of view, only small percentage of women with adult female acne (AFA) has hyperandrogenism. When present, hirsutism, alopecia, change of voice timbre, irregularity of the menstrual cycle, and infertility are the associated features. For such patients, authors suggest endocrine evaluation with free and total testosterone, DHEAS, luteinizing hormone, follicular-stimulating hormone serum dosages, and transvaginal ultrasound of the ovaries. These tests should be performed between 1st and 5th day of menstrual cycle in the morning, between 8:00 and 10:00 am. With these tests, polycystic ovary syndrome (PCOS) is the most frequently associated cause detected. Virilizing tumors and congenital adrenal hyperplasia are the rare causes. However, majority of patients with isolated AFA are found to be normoandrogenic.

In adult women, the lesions are predominantly inflammatory, with mild-to-moderate intensity, tending to be located in the lower third of the face (mandibular line, perioral region). They have increased sensitivity of the skin with higher incidence of postinflammatory erythema, hyper- and/or hypopigmentation, and scarring. Predominant comedo and macrocomedo in the frontal and side regions of the face are reported in smokers over 40 years. Studies show that adult acne has a negative influence on quality of life (QoL), along with signs and symptoms of depression, anxiety and low self-esteem.

Treatment modalities are almost same as for adolescent acne with added hormonal therapy in severe cases. Mild cases can be managed with topical retinoid, azelaic acid, and benzoyl peroxide with or without topical antibiotics. Monotherapy with topical antibiotic is to be avoided to prevent bacterial resistance. Inflammatory lesions respond well to tetracycline group of oral antibiotics. Low-dose oral isotretinoin is preferred, as these patients have increased mucocutaneous sensitivity and may present with irritation.

Hormonal treatments, with combined estrogens with dose between 20 µg and 35 µg and new antiandrogenic progestins, can be used by women when additional contraception is required. They reduce free testosterone levels through an increase of sex hormone-binding globulin (SHBG), a reduction of gonadotropin release, a decrease of ovarian production, and an antiandrogenic effect on sebaceous gland receptors. Apart from improvement of acne, oral contraceptives have added advantage of the reduction of dysmenorrhea, protection against ovary and endometrium cancer, anemia caused by iron deficiency and pelvic inflammatory disease. Nausea, headache, breast pain, sporadic bleeding and decreased libido are the frequent side effects observed with these drugs. Though risk of venous thromboembolism is least in young women, it should be kept in mind.

Studies also show that spironolactone is an aldosterone antagonist effective in the management of adult acne. Menstrual irregularities are the common side effect observed. Monitoring of potassium levels are recommended while on spironolactone.

Key Messages
- Adult acne can be due to persistence of adolescent acne or occurrence at later age
- It predominantly involves lower face and neck
- Adult acne is associated with endocrine abnormalities in very few patients.

ARTICLE 26

Acne: A Side Effect of Masculinizing Hormonal Therapy in Transgender Patients

Motosko CC, Zakhem GA, Pomeranz MK, et al. Acne: a side-effect of masculinizing hormonal therapy in transgender patients.
Br J Dermatol. 2019;180(1):26-30.

Abstract

This article reviews the literature on acne as a side effect of masculinizing hormonal therapy with testosterone in transgender patients. It also highlights the treatment modalities, the precautions to be taken while treating with anti acne therapies, the expected complications of therapy, and how treatment differs in transgender as compared to cisgender.

COMMENT

Masculinizing hormonal treatment with testosterone has been used in transgender men to improve the internal feeling of masculinity, to promote the development of masculine secondary sexual characteristics, and to improve societal perceptions of these patients as male, which in turn brings sense of safety, self-confidence, and symptoms of gender dysphoria in them. However, there are no fixed or standard guidelines for this hormonal therapy.

Testosterone being an androgen acts on the androgen receptors of the sebocytes and mediates sebocyte proliferation. Increased sebum production plays a principal role in the pathogenesis of acne vulgaris. The differential expression of androgen receptors is thought to mediate the distribution of acne lesions. In contrast to U-zones, T-zones of the facial skin express higher levels of androgen receptor protein, which explains the distribution of acne observed clinically. Various studies have shown that number of facial acne and truncal acne increase after starting of masculinizing hormonal therapy. They usually increase within first 4 months then gradually increase over 1 year followed by reduction in some and persistence in few individuals. Acne tends to be most prominent on the back and chest. Dermatologists should be aware of this entity. However, these studies failed to demonstrate correlation between lesion severity and serum levels of luteinizing hormone, testosterone, dihydrotestosterone, estradiol or sex hormone-binding globulin thus highlighting the variable end organ response.

Treatment of acne in transgender is similar to cisgender with topical therapies and systemic antibiotics as a first line of treatment. However, these treatments may be insufficient for complete treatment of androgen-induced acne lesions, and escalation of treatment is often required. Isotretinoin is an important treatment option in treatment failures or may be used as a first-line therapy in patients with severe acne. It acts by antagonizing testosterone effect by diminishing sebocyte proliferation and differentiation, resulting in atrophy and decreased sebum production thus reducing acne.

Hormonal therapy with low-dose ethinylestradiol in combination with either norgestimate, norethindrone or drospirenone, which are used in cisgender for treatment of hormonal acne, should be cautiously used in these patients. However, in authors' experience, it is rare for transgenders to accept these treatment options. If at all if planned it should be given after masculinizing effects of hormonal therapy have reached their maximal effect, which may not occur for more than 2 years after the initiation of testosterone.

Other concern about these patients is risk of hepatotoxicity due to combined toxicity of testosterone, isotretinoin and tetracycline used in the management of acne. Cholestatic jaundice, peliosis hepatis and hematoma are the reported side effects in literature.

Though current evidence does not support the association between isotretinoin and depression, treating physician should monitor for these signs and symptoms as per se transgender may have pre-existing depression. The other side effect is teratogenicity in transgender men who are of childbearing potential, i.e. having ovaries and a uterus. The author suggests that they should be registered as females under iPLEDGE and prescribed accordingly with regular pregnancy test as per the guidelines.

Patients on isotretinoin, if posted for surgery like chest reconstruction, total hysterectomy, salpingo-oophorectomy, vaginectomy, urethroplasty, scrotoplasty, metoidioplasty, and/or phalloplasty, have risk of delayed wound healing and keloid should be considered. Chest binding used by transgenders may increase the truncal acne due to occlusive effect.

> **Key Messages**
> - Transgender on hormonal treatment are prone for acne predominantly in lower face and side of the neck
> - First line of treatment is same as cisgenders with acne and isotretinoin is effective in resistant cases
> - Hormonal treatment, if considered, should be started after masculinizing effects are fully reached.

ARTICLE 27

Efficacy and Safety Profile of Spironolactone 50 mg v/s Isotretinoin 10 mg in the Treatment of Female Patients with Acne Vulgaris Grade 1-2—A Double Blinded, Randomized Comparative Study

Vijayendran N, Kale M, Jamale V, et al. Efficacy and Safety Profile of Spironolactone 50 mg v/s Isotretinoin 10 mg in the Treatment of Female Patients with Acne Vulgaris Grade 1-2—A Double Blinded, Randomized Comparative Study. *JMSCR. 2018;6(2):166-78.*

Abstract

This article determines the safety and efficacy of two treatment modalities, oral isotretinoin and spironolactone for acne vulgaris grade 1-2, and provides standardized data regarding spironolactone as a treatment agent in acne vulgaris. It was observed that isotretinoin is superior to spironolactone in the management of acne. Both the drugs were relatively safe with few side effects like cheilitis with isotretinoin and menstrual irregularities with spironolactone.

COMMENT

Acne predominantly being a disease of adolescents can sometimes persist beyond adolescence or start at a later stage leading to significant psychological impact. Among the various treatment modalities, antiandrogen therapies are also described in literature. This article analyzes safety and efficacy of spironolactone in the management of acne in comparison with oral isotretinoin.

In this randomized, prospective, double blinded, controlled comparative study, subjects were allocated randomly into two groups. Group 1 received tablet isotretinoin 10 mg with topical clindamycin 1%, and group 2 received spironolactone 50 mg/day with topical clindamycin 1% for total 12 weeks. Subjects were assessed every fortnight for efficacy variables with clinical photographs and safety variables. Efficacy variables analysis using Global Acne Grading System (GAGS) score, Physicians Global Assessment (PGA), and Visual Analogue Scale (VAS) showed that at the end of the study (90 days), both groups were efficacious in reducing the PGA and VAS score in acne vulgaris grade 1, 2. However, group 1 with isotretinoin showed statistically significant improvement in GAGS, PGA and VAS as compared to oral spironolactone group.

Clinical improvement was observed from 2nd week in both groups with improvement over 12 weeks. However, isotretinoin group showed accelerated response after 1 month of treatment. In isotretinoin group, improvement of acne lesions with clinically inflammatory papules and comedones was noted all over the face with no site predilection; however in spironolactone group, an improvement of clinically inflammatory papules, which were located predominantly on the lower half of the face and anterior-lateral neck region as compared to lesions, which were comedogenic and present over the forehead and nose.

Safety analysis showed that both drugs were safe with minimal side effects. Cheilitis was the common side effects observed in isotretinoin group and menstrual irregularities like spot bleeding and amenorrhea and less commonly transient diuresis were noted in spironolactone group. Headache was common to both groups.

Key Messages

- Isotretinoin and spironolactone both are efficacious in the treatment of acne vulgaris (grade 1-2); however, isotretinoin is more efficacious than spironolactone
- Spironolactone shows an improvement in clinically inflammatory lesions which are located predominantly on the lower half of the face and anterior-lateral neck region and works better in hyperandrogenic women.

ARTICLE 28

The Microbiome in Preadolescent Acne: Assessment and Prospective Analysis of the Influence of Benzoyl Peroxide

Ahluwalia J, Borok J, Haddock ES, et al. The microbiome in preadolescent acne: Assessment and prospective analysis of the influence of benzoyl peroxide.
Pediatr Dermatol. 2019;36(2):200-6.

Abstract

This study analyzes the microbiome characteristics in preadolescent females with acne vulgaris and the impact of benzoyl peroxide on the microbiome. The microbiome analysis done at baseline and 6–8 weeks after benzoyl peroxide wash using 16S ribosomal RNA (16S rRNA) gene amplicon sequencing showed that microbiome diversity significantly changes with increasing age and number of acne lesions. Higher concentrations of *Cutibacterium acne* (*C. acnes*) were found on forehead and nose than cheeks and chin, and it failed to show significant bacterial diversity (alpha diversity) of the skin at baseline and after treatment with benzoyl peroxide.

COMMENT

Acne being a chronic inflammatory condition has diverse etiology, among which bacterial infection with *Cutibacterium acnes* has received greater attention. It is a normal inhabitant of human skin and sebaceous follicles. Its count is known to increase during puberty and in inflammatory lesion. Though treatment with benzoyl peroxide is known to reduce the quantity of *C. acnes*, its role in establishing microfloral balance has not been studied in detail.

This article aims to throw light on the microbiota characteristics in preadolescent acne patients and effect of benzoyl peroxide on the same. Preadolescent girls between 7 years and 12 years were enrolled for the study. Skin samples were taken from forehead, cheeks, nose, chin, and left retro-auricular crease, and extruded contents of a comedonal lesion were analyzed for microbiota using 16S ribosomal RNA (*16S rRNA*) gene amplicon sequencing on all swab and lesional extraction samples. Repeat tests were done at the end of 6–8 weeks after using benzoyl peroxide 4% wash.

The analysis showed that there was abundance of *C. acnes* in forehead and nose (sebaceous area) as compared to chin and cheeks (nonsebaceous area). There was increase in *C. acnes* with increasing age. This may be attributed to sebaceous gland maturation and increasing sebum secretion. Similarly, statistical increase in *C. acnes* and decrease in *Streptococcus mitis* (*S. mitis*) were observed as the number of acne increased.

It is a well-established fact that benzoyl peroxide exhibits both comedolytic and anti-microbial activity and is lethal to cutaneous organisms, such as *C. acnes*, with varying sensitivities. However in this study, though there was significant reduction in acne lesion after using benzoyl peroxide, it failed to demonstrate significant change in microbiota diversity before and after using benzoyl peroxide wash. The reason may be because of small sample size and collection of sample from stratum corneum instead of the follicular unit. The other possibilities are sampling being done 12 hours after the wash and instead of leave on preparation wash was used.

> **Key Messages**
> - Progressing pubertal maturation is correlated with microbiome shifts
> - An increasing number C. acnes and decrease in S. mitis were noted as the age and number of acne lesions increased
> - Benzoyl peroxide wash failed to demonstrate alteration in microbiota diversity before and after treatment.

ARTICLE 29

Association of Systemic Antibiotic Treatment of Acne with Skin Microbiota Characteristics

Chien AL, Tsai J, Leung S, et al. Association of Systemic Antibiotic Treatment of Acne with Skin Microbiota Characteristics. *JAMA Dermatol.* 2019. [Epub ahead of print]

Abstract
Antibiotics are one of the frequently prescribed drugs in the management of acne. Rampant and prolonged use of antibiotics changes complete bacterial community of the skin. This article explores the composition, diversity and resilience of skin microbiota in acne patients on systemic antibiotics.

COMMENT

Acne being a chronic inflammatory disorder of pilosebaceous unit is regularly managed with systemic antibiotics. This longitudinal cohort study aims to establish the effect of these antibiotics on the composition of microbiota of the skin. The study involved acne patients who were treated with doxycycline 100 mg twice daily for 4 weeks. Skin areas on the forehead, cheek and chin were sampled for 16S ribosomal RNA (*16S rRNA*) gene sequencing at baseline, 4 weeks after starting antibiotic treatment, and then

1 week and 8 weeks after discontinuation of treatment. Skin microbiota was examined with respect to relative abundance and diversity of bacterial taxa. The analysis of data showed that postantibiotic treatment, a 1.4-fold reduction in the level of *Cutibacterium acnes* (*C. acnes*), which recovered following cessation of treatment. There was transient increase in *Pseudomonas* species count by 5.6-fold immediately following antibiotic treatment along with persistent 1.7-fold increase in *Streptococcus* species count. 4.7-fold decrease was noted in *Lactobacillus* species 8 weeks following antibiotic treatment withdrawal. In conclusion, it was observed that, antibiotic administration was associated with an initial alteration from baseline of bacterial diversity followed by recovery. Understanding the association between systemic antibiotic use and skin microbiota may help clinicians to decrease the likelihood of skin comorbidities related to microbial dysbiosis. Systemic antibiotic treatment may reduce bacterial populations beneficial to skin health like *Lactobacillus* species, which may predispose to skin infections. These data stress the importance of concurrent monitoring of the skin microbiota during antibiotic therapy, a need for targeted antibiotic therapies, or additional therapies to retain the "good" flora during treatment.

Key Messages
- Systemic antibiotics alter the microbiota of the skin by reducing C. acnes levels
- At the same time, it may alter good flora like Lactobacillus thus making prone for infections
- So, targeted antibiotic therapy is the need of the hour.

ARTICLE 30

Novel Nicotinamide Skin-adhesive Hot Melt Extrudates for Treatment of Acne

Nasr M, Karandikar H, Abdel-Aziz RT, et al. Novel nicotinamide skin-adhesive hot melt extrudates for treatment of acne. *Expert Opin Drug Deliv.* 2018;15(12):1165-73.

Abstract
The aim of this study was to prepare, characterize and explore the applicability of medicated hot melt extrudates based on nicotinamide and Soluplus polymer, in acne treatment. The extrudates were also tested for their skin adhesion potential, ability to deposit nicotinamide in different skin layers, and the clinical efficacy of these extrudates was also tested. The 10% nicotinamide extrudates exhibited amorphous nature which was reserved during storage, with no chemical

interaction between nicotinamide and Soluplus. Also, these extrudates displayed significantly higher adhesion and drug deposition reaching 4.8-folds, 5.3-folds and 4.3-folds more in the stratum corneum, epidermis and dermis, respectively. The total number of acne lesions was significantly reduced by 61.3% in extrudates compared to 42.14% with the nicotinamide gel.

Conclusion: Soluplus extrudates are promising topical drug delivery means for the treatment of dermatological diseases.

COMMENT

Hot melt extrusion is a pharmaceutical technique for production of uniform dispersions of drugs within polymeric matrices. This is environment-friendly due to the lack of solvent use. Soluplus is a polymer that has been reported to create solid solutions. Soluplus is a graft copolymer composed of poly(N-vinyl caprolactam/vinyl acetate/ethylene glycol), which due to its amphiphilicity is used as a surfactant to solubilize poorly soluble drugs. When this is used with another agent in topical agent, the contact extrudates with the skin creates an occlusive condition, which enhances the delivery of the drug.

Topical application of nicotinamide stabilizes the epidermal barrier function and decreases the transepidermal water loss from the stratum corneum. Its mechanism in acne is by decreasing the rate of sebum excretion, inhibitory effect on *Propionibacterium acnes*, and its anti-inflammatory effects. As it is hydrophilic, it is a challenge to deliver adequate amounts of nicotinamide to the skin.

Patients were instructed to apply a thin film of the nicotinamide gel on the left half of the face once daily (at an amount which is sufficient to cover the acne lesion), and selected nicotinamide extrudate on the right side of the face once daily after wetting an extrudate patch (of dimension 1 cm × 1 cm) with two drops of water using a dropper. Patients were instructed to press the wetted side of the extrudate firmly onto the skin for 30 seconds. The treatment period was continued up to 8 weeks. All patients were photographed every 2 weeks, and evaluated clinically at the end of the 8 weeks through the counting of comedones, inflammatory and total acne lesions at both sides of the by 2-blinded dermatologists. Nicotinamide Soluplus extrudates significantly reduced the total number of acne lesions as compared to the nicotinamide side. Skin adhesion and deposition studies demonstrated that Soluplus was able to adhere to the skin creating a film that was able to deposit nicotinamide in all skin layers. The bioadhesive property exhibited by the prepared extrudates is desirable from both the pharmaceutical and clinical points of view, since they act as a drug reservoir providing sustained release of nicotinamide. No adverse effects were noted.

Key Message

- *Soluplus extrudates are promising topical drug delivery means for the treatment of dermatological diseases.*

ARTICLE 31

Treatment of Acne with a Combination of Propolis, Tea Tree Oil and *Aloe vera* Compared to Erythromycin Cream: Two Double-blind Investigations

Mazzarello V, Donadu MG, Ferrari M, et al. Treatment of acne with a combination of propolis, tea tree oil, and *Aloe vera* compared to erythromycin cream: two double-blind investigations.
Clin Pharmacol: Adv Appl. 2018;10:175.

Abstract

Topical antibiotics are often prescribed as the first-line therapy for acne. The efficacy of topical antibiotics is becoming less effective due to the development of antibiotic resistance. This study aimed to evaluate the anti-acne efficacy of a new cream based on three natural extracts of propolis, tea tree oil and *Aloe vera*, comparing it to erythromycin cream and placebo. Sixty patients with mild-to-moderate acne were randomly divided into three groups and treated with cream containing 20% propolis, 3% tea tree oil, and 10% *Aloe vera* (PTAC), or with 3% erythromycin cream (ERC); or with placebo. The lesions were assessed at baseline, 15 days and 30 days by acne lesional count. All the clinical and instrumental values studied were statistically different from placebo except for sebometry, pH metry, and erythema index values, measured on healthy skin. Unlike in the placebo group, papular and scar lesions showed high erythema reduction after 15 and 30 days of PTAC and ERC application.

Conclusion: The PTAC formulation was better than ERC in reducing erythema scars, acne severity index, and total lesion count.

COMMENT

Acne is a common disorder, though not a serious life-threatening illness, acne and the scarring results in significant psychological morbidity. Acne has various pathogenetic mechanisms. Different therapeutic agents target different mechanisms. Mild-to-moderate acne is usually treated with topical antibiotics, retinoids and benzoyl peroxide. There is a risk of development of resistance with topical antibiotics, so it should not be prescribed as a monotherapy for acne. Addition of a retinoid or benzoyl peroxide reduced the risk of development of resistance. This study was performed to evaluate the efficacy of a new cream based on three natural extracts (propolis, tea tree oil, and *Aloe vera*) in treating mild-to-moderate acne, comparing it to a cream based on 3% erythromycin and to its vehicle alone (placebo).

Sixty patients with mild-to-moderate acne were included in the study and randomized to receive each of the above therapy. Propolis is known to have antibacterial effects, more toward gram-positive bacteria. It is bacteriostatic at low concentrations and bactericidal at high concentrations. The tea tree oil contains several monoterpenes, and the most abundant of these is terpinen-4-ol. Multiple earlier studies have shown the effectiveness of tea tree oil in reducing mild acne. The average minimal inhibitory concentration of tea tree oil against *P. acnes* and *S. epidermidis* was in the range between 0.31% and 0.63% v/v. The minimum bactericidal concentration, required to eliminate *P. acnes*, was 0.5% v/v. *Aloe vera* is known to have anti-inflammatory and anti-acne properties. All the clinical tools showed a considerable reduction in acne with the two groups as compared to placebo. The PTAC formulation was better than ERC in reducing erythema scars, thus speeding up healing time, as early as the first 15 days of treatment. The PTAC was more effective in reducing erythema scars. The papular erythema reduction was similar in the PTAC and ERC group. The sebometry, pH metry and erythema index values, measured on healthy skin, did not undergo statistically significant changes during the treatment in the three study groups. PTAC was found to be more effective in reducing the acne severity index. No side effects were noted.

> **Key Message**
> - In the era of growing antibiotic resistance, alternate therapies for acne should be explored. This study shows that combination of propolis, tea tree oil and Aloe vera is effective in mild-to-moderate acne.

ARTICLE 32

The Safety and Efficacy of Four Different Fixed Combination Regimens of Adapalene 0.1%/Benzoyl Peroxide 2.5% Gel for the Treatment of Acne Vulgaris: Results from a Randomized Controlled Study

Tan J, Bissonnette R, Gratton D, et al. The safety and efficacy of four different fixed combination regimens of adapalene 0.1%/benzoyl peroxide 2.5% gel for the treatment of acne vulgaris: results from a randomized controlled study. *Eur J Dermatol. 2018;28(4):502-8.*

Abstract

Fixed combination of adapalene 0.1%/benzoyl peroxide 2.5% gel (A/BPO) is recommended as a topical therapy for acne. Because of the tolerability issues, patient adherence is compromised, thus affecting the treatment outcome. This multicentric single-blinded controlled study was designed to determine whether modified adapalene/benzoyl peroxide regimens improve tolerability during the first 4 weeks of treatment without impairing the clinical response. About 120 patients with mild-to-moderate acne were included in the study who received, during the first 4 weeks, A/BPO daily overnight (A/BPO-EN), A/BPO daily for 3 hours (A/BPO-3h), A/BPO daily overnight and a provided moisturizer lotion (A/BPO-moisturizer), or A/BPO every other night (A/BPO-EoN). The assessment was done for local tolerance, global worst score (GWS), and total sum score (TSS). Efficacy was assessed based on lesion counts, investigator global assessment (IGA), and total lesion count reduction. The mean TSS was significantly reduced at first week with A/BPO-EoN versus A/BPO-EN ($p < 0.05$), and A/BPO-EoN led to the lowest GWS and a decrease in severity of stinging/burning and erythema ($p < 0.05$). Dryness and scaling were less in the A/BPO-moisturizer regimen compared with the A/BPO-EN regimen. The median decrease in lesions from baseline was similar in all groups—up to 67% for total, 72% for inflammatory and 70% for noninflammatory lesion counts. Adherence, IGA, patient satisfaction, and overall safety were excellent.

Conclusion: Modulating treatment regimens during the first 4 weeks improved local tolerability without impacting overall efficacy outcome after 12 weeks and may improve treatment adherence during the first weeks of therapy.

COMMENT

As acne vulgaris is multifactorial, combination therapies are recommended. The most commonly used combination is that of topical retinoid and benzoyl peroxide. Fixed dose combination of adapalene 0.1%/benzoyl peroxide 2.5% gel is a rational choice due to the complementary action of both the agents. There are many reports which have proved the efficacy of this combination as a monotherapy. It has also been reported that the combination acts much faster and effectively than each drug alone. Patient tolerability is a concern with this combination. Both agents cause skin dryness and redness. If patients do not tolerate the medicine, then there will be difficulty in adherence which results in noneffective treatment. Physicians normally give a modified regimen especially in the first 2 weeks to allow skin adaptation. Commonly used regimens are the shorter duration of application or reduced frequency. In this study, the various different regimens were compared. Four different regimens were used, A/BPO daily overnight, A/BPO daily for 3 hour, A/BPO daily overnight and a provided moisturizer lotion, and A/BPO every other night. At the end of 4 weeks, A/BPO daily overnight and a moisturizer lotion group had significantly less scaling and dryness. The stinging and burning sensation was less with the A/BPO every other night group. Clinical efficacy at the end of 12 weeks was similar in all groups. Using the above modifications helps to reduce the side effects of the fixed drug combination leading to better compliance.

Key Message

- Modifications of fixed combination adapalene 0.1%/benzoyl peroxide 2.5% gel regimens like A/BPO daily overnight and a moisturizer lotion, and A/BPO every other night reduces the side effects, increases tolerability and patient adherence.

ARTICLE 33

Survey of Acne-related Post-inflammatory Hyperpigmentation in the Middle East

Abanmi A, Al-Enezi M, Al Hammadi A, et al. Survey of acne-related post-inflammatory hyperpigmentation in the Middle East.
J Dermatol Treat. 2018:1-4.

Abstract

Acne vulgaris is a very common inflammatory skin disease in the Middle East, similar to other regions of the world. Majority of the population in the Middle East is of darker pigmentation (Fitzgerald skin types III-VI). Skin of color is more prone to develop post-inflammatory hyperpigmentation (PIH) as a sequela of acne. PIH was present in 87.2% of subjects in this prospective noninterventional study of acne patients consulting dermatologists (n = 262) in the Middle East. The majority of subjects (52.6%) reported that PIH had been present for 1 year or longer. About 69.0% of subjects gave history of excoriating their acne lesions, suggesting that this may be a major modifiable risk factor for physicians to stress during patient education efforts. Half of the subjects indicated that PIH was more bothersome than acne.

COMMENT

Post-inflammatory pigmentation of acne is more in the skin of color. In this review, the authors have surveyed post-inflammatory hyperpigmentation (PIH) and the treatment. This study was done among the Middle East population. A significant proportion of the acne patient populations in Middle Eastern countries tend to have moderate to darkly pigmented skin and are at high risk for PIH as a sequela to acne. PIH presents as localized or diffuse colored macules in previous sites of acne. In the early stages, the pigmentation may be masked by erythema, and the pigmentation becomes more prominent as the treatment ensues.

In this study, they found that 87% of subjects had PIH. Seventy percent had moderate PIH and the remaining severe PIH, with the pigmentation being present for more than a year. Sixty-nine percent gave a history of manipulation of the acne lesions.

Post-inflammatory hyperpigmentation also is significantly worrisome to the patient as acne. While treating patients we should counsel them about the risk of hyperpigmentation especially in skin types IV to VI. Other than the skin color, picking or manipulation of acne (acne excoriee) is a risk factor for pigmentation. The primary strategy for treatment of PIH is sun protection, early treatment of acne and counseling. Topical retinoids, fixed combinations of retinoids with benzoyl peroxide, salicylic acid peels and glycolic acid peels, Kligman's formula and its modifications are the various treatment options available.

> **Key Message**
> ⦿ Acne-associated PIH is common among patients with the skin of color. Early treatment of acne, sunscreen and counseling help to prevent it to some extent.

ARTICLE 34

The Use of Hormonal Antiandrogen Therapy in Female Patients with Acne: A 10-year Retrospective Study

Park JH, Bienenfeld A, Orlow SJ, et al. The use of hormonal antiandrogen therapy in female patients with acne: a 10-year retrospective study.
Am J Clin Dermatol. 2018;19(3):449-55.

Abstract

The aim of this study was to investigate the prescribing pattern of hormonal antiandrogen acne treatment (HAAT) by dermatologists for acne. In this retrospective study, female patients receiving HAAT was studied over a period of 10 years. Data from a control group of female acne patients who never received HAAT were also collected. It was found that systemic antibiotics were the most common medications, followed by spironolactone and then oral contraceptive pills. Mean antibiotic durations in patients who initiated HAAT for the first time at the study site (250.4 days) were significantly longer than in patients who received HAAT prior to presentation and continued HAAT at the study site (192.0 days). A statistically significant inverse association was found between HAAT use and mean antibiotic duration.

Conclusion: HAAT is not typically associated with shorter cumulative antibiotic durations and early HAAT initiation can decrease systemic antibiotic use in acne treatment.

COMMENT

Acne is a common chronic disorder of pilosebaceous glands. Systemic antibiotics and retinoids are the common systemic agents prescribed in moderate-to-severe acne. Though acne is common among boys, adult acne is more common in women. In women antiandrogen therapy is also a systemic therapy option. Hormonal antiandrogen acne treatment (HAAT) can be prescribed to all women with acne, even those with normal hormonal profile, and no overt signs of hyperandrogenism. HAAT used to treat acne include combined oral contraceptives (COCs), spironolactone, and less commonly, estrogen and flutamide.

In this retrospective study of 10 years, 3,996 female patients with acne were identified. About 672 patients were prescribed HAAT. About 222 patients (33.0%) had acne in the chin or perioral region, 223 patients (33.2%) on the cheeks, 193 (28.7%) on the forehead, and 114 (16.9%) on the jawline. About 211 patients (31.4%) had perimenstrual acne flares, 49 patients (7.3%) had hirsutism, and 49 patients (7.3%) had irregular menses. About 411 patients (61.2%) were treated with COCs, 197 patients (29.3%) were treated with spironolactone, and 64 patients (9.5%) were treated with COCs and spironolactone, simultaneously or at different times.

It was noted that only 44.4% of dermatologists who prescribed COCs for acne documented discussion of COC risks and side effects. HAAT was the second- or third-line therapy in acne. Earlier studies have reported that though antibiotics are effective in reducing inflammatory lesions early, by 6 months both HAAT and antibiotics have similar efficacy.

> **Key Message**
> - The HAAT is an effective and well-tolerated therapy for inflammatory acne in adult women. It can be used as an alternative to systemic antibiotics as the first line of therapy.

ARTICLE 35

Adapalene 0.3% Gel Shows Efficacy for the Treatment of Atrophic Acne Scars

Loss MJ, Leung S, Chien A, et al. Adapalene 0.3% gel shows efficacy for the treatment of atrophic acne scars. *Dermatol Ther. 2018;8(2):245-57.*

Abstract

Acne scarring causes a lot of psychological morbidity in the individual. Current therapies for acne scars are mainly surgical and laser therapy. These may not be affordable by all patients. Here, the authors have evaluated a higher concentration of adapalene gel, i.e. 0.3% in management of atrophic acne scars. They have noted an improvement of 50% in skin texture and about 80% improvement in acne scars. The drug was well-tolerated by most patients.

COMMENT

Acne vulgaris is a common chronic condition affecting the pilosebaceous glands. The prevalence is about 80% in adolescence. Acne scarring, which is an unfortunate sequela of acne, causes significant psychological morbidity. Acne scars result from delay in treatment or inadequate treatment and healing of inflammatory lesions. Atrophic acne scars are the most common types of acne scars. The currently available treatment options for acne scars are mainly nonpharmacological and invasive like surgery, dermabrasion, fillers and laser devices. These are expensive and not all patients will be able to afford it. Topical therapies which are effective in acne scarring are sparse as the damage is at the level of the dermis.

Topical retinoids have been approved for the management of acne and photodamaged skin. The ability of retinoids to stimulate dermal fibroblasts to increase the production of procollagen is well established. Adapalene 0.3% gel is approved for the management of acne. It is also used in actinic keratosis, solar lentigenes and photodamaged skin. As the effect of adapalene on photodamaged skin and fine wrinkles is by collagen stimulation, the authors speculated its use in atrophic acne scars.

Patients with atrophic acne scars were enrolled in the study and prescribed once daily application of adapalene 0.3% for 4 weeks, and twice daily for the next 20 weeks. Additional cleansers, moisturizers and sunscreens were given to the patients as well. Patients were assessed regularly till week 72. Biopsy was also done from a few patients to ascertain any molecular alterations that may explain potential clinical improvement. Standard immunohistochemistry methods were used to examine the expression levels of dermal matrix molecules, including Procol-1 and Procol-3.

By week 24 about 55% of patients showed improvement in acne scars assessed by full-face global scarring grade. The scarring continued to improve even after patients stopped treatment. According to subject global assessment scale improvement in skin texture and acne scars was seen in 83% and 89% of patients. In terms of dermal matrix macromolecules, both type I collagen alpha 1 (COL1A1) and type III collagen alpha 1 (COL3A1) showed higher expression.

Key Message

- Daily use of adapalene 0.3% gel for the treatment of atrophic acne scars showed promising clinical efficacy, a favorable tolerability profile and improvement in quality of life.

ARTICLE 36

Evaluation the Efficacy of Trichloroacetic Acid 33% in Treatment of Oral Retinoid-induced Cheilitis Compared with Placebo (Vaseline): A Randomized Pilot Study

Mansouri P, Azizian Z, Hejazi S, et al. Evaluation the efficacy of trichloroacetic acid (TCA) 33% in treatment of oral retinoid-induced cheilitis compared with placebo (vaseline): a randomized pilot study.
J Dermatol Treat. 2018;29(7):694-7.

Abstract

Isotretinoin is currently the most effective and commonly used medication to treat moderate-to-severe acne. The most common side effect of isotretinoin is cheilitis. In this study, the authors have studied the efficacy of trichloroacetic acid (TCA) 33% in comparison to Vaseline in the management of cheilitis. They have reported TCA to be more effective than placebo in cheilitis.

COMMENT

Isotretinoin is considered as the gold standard in the management of moderate-to-severe acne vulgaris. The most common side effect of isotretinoin is chelitis. The absence of chelitis is also used as a marker for drug noncompliance. A study has reported that chelitis occurs in about 78% of the patients on isotretinoin and is also the most common cause for discontinuation of therapy. Cheilitis causes lot of discomfort to the patient. Trichloroacetic acid is a strong water-soluble acid and absorbs air humidity. The authors have used low concentration of trichloroacetic acid (TCA) to treat patients with cheilitis. Trichloroacetic acid induces precipitation of proteins and coagulative necrosis of epidermis and upper dermal layers. This facilitates collagen remodeling and re-epithelialization.

Ninety patients who had cheilitis due to isotretinoin were randomized into two groups for therapy with TCA 33% and placebo (Vaseline). Single application of TCA was done in the clinic and for controls, Vaseline was asked to be applied twice daily. They were reviewed at 2 and 6 weeks for improvement in the lesions. At the end of 6 weeks, there was a significant reduction in erythema in the TCA group, however, reduction in scaling and crusting was similar in both groups.

Cheilitis is treated with emollients and a short course of topical steroids when severe. In this study, other than the improvement in erythema, TCA was not found to be more effective than TCA. But the advantage is the single application of TCA, as compared to the daily application of petroleum jelly. The authors have not noted any side effects with TCA application.

> **Key Message**
> - A combination treatment with single application of TCA 33% with Vaseline petroleum jelly regularly can be an effective option in the management of cheilitis due to isotretinoin.

ARTICLE 37

Light Therapies for Acne: Abridged Cochrane Systematic Review including GRADE Assessments

Barbaric J, Abbott R, Posadzki P, et al. Light therapies for acne: abridged Cochrane systematic review including GRADE assessments.
Br J Dermatol. 2018;178(1):61-75.

Abstract

The article is a Cochrane systematic review evaluating the safety and efficacy of light-based interventions for acne vulgaris (AV). It reviewed randomized controlled trials (RCTs) under Cochrane Skin Specialized Register, CENTRAL, MEDLINE, Embase, LILACS, ISI Web of Science, and grey literature sources. Various articles comparing different light based studies showed that none of these modalities showed significant improvement in acne lesions. Side effects like blistering were noted in few. Further research is required in this field.

COMMENT

Acne is a common disorder affecting pilosebaceous unit with various treatment options like topical medications, systemic agents, procedure-based and light-based treatments, each having its own pros and cons with respect to safety and efficacy. Light therapies utilize light with different properties like wavelength, intensity, coherent or incoherent light. Though their exact mode of action is not known, three factors important in therapeutic outcome are light, photosensitizers, and oxidative stress. Photosensitizers can be endogenous, that is porphyrins produced by *P. acnes* or exogenous as in photodynamic therapy (PDT) which uses 5-aminolevulinic acid (5-ALA) and its methyl-ester methyl-aminolevulinate (MAL). These photosensitizers absorb light to form a highly reactive singlet oxygen species which damage bacteria and sebocytes due to oxidative stress. Interference with the immunological response is another proposed mechanism of action with PDT.

The article analyzed 71 articles involving 4,211 participants undergoing various light therapies. In two studies comparing yellow light with placebo or no treatment showed conflicting results with one study showing no difference in results between yellow light treated and placebo group while others showed improvement in acne count. Thus, authors could not confirm the results. Two other split face studies comparing efficacy of Infrared light (1450 nm laser) and Nd: YAG laser with placebo showed reduction in mainly inflammatory lesions as compared to noninflammatory lesions on treated side as compared to placebo. Another split face study with Fractional Erbium Glass Laser, found statistically significant reduction in both inflammatory and noninflammatory lesions.

Blue light has shown promising results in various studies with significant differences in mean percentage improvements in both inflammatory and noninflammatory lesions at final treatment. In another study comparing blue light with topical benzoyl peroxide (BPO) mean reduction was observed in noninflammatory group in both the groups however, data regarding inflammatory lesions was not available. However, another split-face study comparing a combination of BPO and three sessions of 530–750 nm light with BPO alone observed no significant difference between light-treated and untreated sides of the face for changes in mean papule and pustule counts.

A study comparing four sessions of red light plus 80 mg/g MAL with placebo cream and red light showed that MAL-PDT was not superior to red light alone in efficacy. However, MAL–PDT versus placebo split face study has shown greater reduction inflammatory acne with MAL-PDT as compared to placebo. However, due to lack of data, authors were unable to confirm results. In another study comparing 80 mg/g MAL-PDT with 40 mg/g MAL-PDT showed no difference in efficacy in both groups.

In a split-face trial comparing three sessions of 20% ALA plus PDL with untreated control showed statistically significant decrease in papule count but no significant difference in pustules, cysts and noninflammatory lesions. Another study comparing different strengths of ALA showed that that 20% ALA was not superior to 15% ALA but was more effective than 10% and 5% ALA. Overall evidence suggests that using lower ALA doses (15% and 10%), together with light modalities other than blue light may be of benefit. This is because several studies found that of 20% ALA had more adverse effects like blistering. Another study showed that Gold micro particle PDT was superior to vehicle.

Thus though this review includes a comprehensive search for all eligible studies, due to limited evidence, authors are unable to draw firm conclusions to guide decisions in practice, especially considering the cost of light-based treatments. Lack of long-term follow-up was the drawback in all studies. More robust, well-planned studies with greater sample sizes comparing the effectiveness of common acne treatments with light therapies are need of the hour.

Key Messages

- *The overall quality of evidence for light-based therapy is very low*
- *A few studies reported blue-red light to be superior to placebo, and blue light to have similar effects as BPO*
- *About 20% ALA-PDT activated by blue light did not show superior effectiveness in comparison with blue light alone thus proving low evidence to suggest as standard line of treatment.*

ARTICLE 38

Dapsone-loaded Invasomes as a Potential Treatment of Acne: Preparation, Characterization and In Vivo Skin Deposition Assay

El-Nabarawi MA, Shamma RN, Farouk F, et al. Dapsone-loaded invasomes as a potential treatment of acne: preparation, characterization, and in vivo skin deposition assay.
AAPS PharmSciTech. 2018;19(5):2174-84.

Abstract

Dapsone is a sulfone antibiotic. It also has strong anti-inflammatory effects, due to which it is used in many indications in dermatology. Topical dapsone has been used in acne vulgaris. In this study, the dapsone loaded invasomes were evaluated to study the deposition assay. It was found that these invasomes helped in better delivery of dapsone through the skin and the concentration of dapsone on the skin was 2.5 times higher than alcoholic dapsone preparation. By invasomes, the drug availability of dapsone through topical application can be enhanced.

COMMENT

Dapsone is a sulfone compound with both antibacterial and anti-inflammatory effects. This combination makes it a good option in the management of acne. Due to the side effects of systemic dapsone on long-term use, topical dapsone is used in the management of acne vulgaris routinely.

Invasomes are vesicles with enhanced percutaneous penetration as compared to liposomes. They are elastic phospholipid vesicles containing phosphatidylcholine, ethanol and terpenes. These terpenes enhance the percutaneous penetration by disrupting stratum corneum lipids and improvement of partition of drugs into stratum corneum. In this study, the ability of invasomes to transport topical dapsone was studied. The ability of the invasome to deliver dapsone to the skin was studied by in vivo and in vitro using Wistar rats. Different formulations of invasomes with various terpenes were tried. Limonene containing terpene invasome showed the best results for enhanced penetration of dapsone in in-vitro techniques. Limonene is highly lipophilic, which is the reason for its enhanced penetration. Increasing the quantity of terpene, resulted in increased absorption of dapsone. In vivo deposition of dapsone was studied in rats. Invasome dapsone had a higher skin deposition profile in comparison to alcohol-based formulation. The skin deposition of the drug was 2.5 times higher with invasome in comparison to the control.

> **Key Message**
>
> - Invasomes with topical dapsone enhance the percutaneous absorption of dapsone. This translates to better clinical efficacy and effective management of acne.

ARTICLE 39

Prevention and Reduction of Atrophic Acne Scars with Adapalene 0.3%/Benzoyl Peroxide 2.5% Gel in Subjects with Moderate or Severe Facial Acne: Results of a 6-month Randomized, Vehicle-controlled Trial using Intra-individual Comparison

Dréno B, Bissonnette R, Gagné-Henley A, et al. Prevention and reduction of atrophic acne scars with adapalene 0.3%/benzoyl peroxide 2.5% gel in subjects with moderate or severe facial acne: results of a 6-month randomized, vehicle-controlled trial using intra-individual comparison.
Am J Clin Dermatol. 2018;19(2):275-86.

Abstract

Acne causes a lot of psychological distress due to its scarring. Scar treatment is usually with surgical methods and lasers. Topical retinoid is also used to mild scarring. In this study, the authors have evaluated the effects of higher concentration of adapalene 0.3% and benzoyl peroxide on atrophic scar formation. In this split-face clinical trial higher concentration of topical adapalene 0.3% and benzoyl peroxide combination considerably reduced the acne count as well as acne scars.

COMMENT

Acne scars are common sequelae of acne. Scarring can be prevented to some extent by early and effective treatment of acne. Among the various types of acne scars, atrophic scars due to loss of collagen are the most common. Scarring in acne is related to the severity of acne, but in susceptible individuals even mild acne can heal with atrophic scars. A wide variety of topical medications are available for acne management. Topical retinoids are the most favored among them as they target almost all the pathogenic mechanisms involved in acne and reduce the formation of microcomedones which are acne precursor lesions. Adapalene a synthetic retinoid is known for its anticomedogenic, keratolytic, anti-inflammatory and immunoregulatory effects. As acne is multifactorial combination therapies will work better than a single agent. In this study, a fixed dose combination of Adapalene 0.3%/benzoyl peroxide 2.5% gel was prescribed to one half of the face and vehicle on the other half was used as control. Benzoyl peroxide has potent antibacterial effect, and unlike topical antibiotics, there is no risk of resistance. It has been shown that the percutaneous absorption of adaplene is enhanced in the combination. Management of acne scars requires surgical procedures and laser therapy. These are time consuming and also a financial burden to the patient. Preventive strategies for acne scars are always better. It is well known that retinoids induce collagen remodeling; adaplene 0.3% has shown to improve the skin texture and atrophic scars as well. This study has shown a significant reduction in the acne count as well as acne scars when a combination therapy was used. Studies with 0.1% adapalene have not shown any reduction in atrophic scar count, in contrast where 0.3% adapalene in this study has shown a 30% reduction in acne scar count.

When using this combination on Indian skin, the side effects are of concern. Both benzoyl peroxide and adapalene cause skin dryness and irritation. With an increased concentration of adapalene the incidence of irritation is bound to be higher, that might reduce the patient compliance and adherence to medication. In this study, two patients have withdrawn from the study due to irritation and pain on the skin.

Key Message
- About 0.3% adapalene though more efficacious in treating acne and preventing acne scars, has a risk of severe irritation and redness on Indian skin.

ARTICLE 40

Complementary and Alternative Methods for Treatment of Acne Vulgaris: A Systematic Review

Marous MR, Flaten HK, Sledge B, et al. Complementary and alternative methods for treatment of acne vulgaris: a systematic review.
Curr Dermatol Rep. 2018;7(4):359-70.

Abstract
Acne is a very common disorder with a prevalence of up to 80% among adolescents. This review compiles the use of alternative medicines on acne vulgaris. Oral green tea extract, nicotinamide both oral and topical and oral zinc have been shown to be effective in the management of acne. More studies are required to study the effects of these alternative methods in comparison to the conventional treatment.

COMMENT

Complementary and alternative medicine (CAM) is the term for medical products and practices that are not part of standard medical care. Some CAM have undergone careful evaluation and have found to be safe and effective. Complementary medications are usually natural and less invasive. CAM is often sought by people who suffer chronic illness, and when conventional therapy is not showing significant clinical improvement in a short time. Also if patients experience any side effects of conventional therapy they go for CAM.

Acne is a chronic disorder and we have a wide array of conventional treatment methods. As it is a chronic disorder patients sometime seek alternate methods of treatment, as it is a popular belief that alternate treatment are natural and have minimal side effects. The authors have reviewed articles on alternate methods of treatment for acne. Many studies in the past have shown beneficial effects of complementary and alternative methods in acne management.

Oral green tea extract has been shown to reduce the amount of sebum and also reduce inflammatory acne lesions in comparison with a placebo. Epigallocatechin-3-gallate (EGCG), the major polyphenol in green tea, has shown to cause a reduction in sebum and inflammation as well as an induction of sebocyte apoptosis and decreased viability of *Propionibacterium acnes*. Thus, all the mechanisms of acne are targeted by this 4% nicotinamide gel has been found to be similar in efficacy to 1% clindamycin and 4% erythromycin. Nicotinamide is available in combination with clindamycin in various acne preparations.

Zinc both topical and oral formulation has not been found to be effective in acne. Studies comparing oral zinc with oral minocycline, showed zinc to have very inferior performance. Ocimum oil is found to be as effective as 1% clindamycin. When used with adapalene, *Ginkgo biloba*/mannitol had an additive effect, the arm of patients using these combinations had a better response than adapalene alone. About 3% cannabis seed extract cream was compared against a vehicle to check for reduction in erythema post acne, and the effect of 3% cannabis was found to be significant in reducing erythema. Other CAM which were found to be effective are cedar wood oil, clay jojoba facial masks, Copaiba essential oil, ginger, honey bee venom, *Hippophae rhamnoides* and *Cassia fistula* plant extract, honeybee venom. However better research and comparative studies are required to further establish these CAM as a definitive therapy for acne. It should be noted that CAM are not completely safe and devoid of side effects.

Key Message

- The CAM helps to reduce the development of resistance with topical antibiotics in acne. Combining these CAM with conventional medicines seems to enhance the effects like addition of nicotinamide to clindamycin, Ginkgo biloba to adapalene, cedar wood oil to tretinoin.

ARTICLE 41

Effects of the Myrtle Essential Oil on the Acne Skin—Clinical Trials for Korean Women

Kim KY, Jang HH, Lee SN, et al. Effects of the myrtle essential oil on the acne skin—clinical trials for Korean women. *Biomed Dermatol. 2018;2(1):28.*

Abstract

This study was conducted to clinically verify the effects of myrtle essential oil, on acne skin of Korean women. The purpose was to develop natural substances with high safety to relieve acne and minimize skin irritation. Subjects were divided into two groups—one was treated with myrtle essential oil applied (the experimental group) and the no-treatment group with no myrtle essential oil applied (the control group). The duration of the study was 6 weeks. All the constituents of the cosmetics were similar except for the presence or absence of myrtle substances, to precisely check the effects of the myrtle substances. The acne grades significantly improved in the experimental group with myrtle applied, with the pore index (outstanding pores, large pores, and blackheads), the erythema index, the sebum index, and the desquamation index also improving. The micro-organism index also decreased considerably in the experimental group. This showed that adding myrtle substances significantly improved acne.

COMMENT

The pathomechanisms in acne involve increased sebum production, hyperkeratinization of dead skin cells, proliferation of *Propionibacterium acnes* and inflammatory reaction. Myrtle essential oil has been used for treating acne, oily skin and loose pores in many cultures. It is known as soft mild oil. Myrtle essential oil comprises 35.9% of myrtenyl acetate, an ester substance; 29.89% of 1,8-cineole, an oxide substance; and 8.18% of a-pinene and 7.58% of limonene, which are monoterpene substances. These ester, oxide, and mono terpene-based substances are presumed to have antibacterial effects and keratinolytic action. The aim of this study was to examine the impacts of myrtle essential oil on Koreans' acne skin and to reveal its possibility to be used for cosmetics for acne-prone skin without causing any irritation. Korean Acne Grading System (KAGS), the erythema index, the pore index, the sebum index, the desquamation index and the micro-organism index was used to identify 20 women with acne-prone skin and divide them into experimental groups and controls.

The control group was asked to use a foam cleanser, toner, emulsion and sunblock none of which contained myrtle substances. On the other hand, the experimental group was given a foam cleanser, toner, emulsion and sunblock containing myrtle substances. Myrtle oil containing group did not experience any side effects. All of the acne grades, the erythema index, the pore index, the desquamation index and the micro-organism index showed an improvement, with a statistically significant result in the experimental group.

> **Key Message**
>
> - This study has clinically proved that myrtle essential oil has effects for reduction in erythema, removal of sebum and antibacterial activity on the facial skin of Korean women. It can be considered to be safe in people with acne-prone skin.

ARTICLE 42

Comparison of Efficacy of Commercially Available versus Freshly Prepared Salicylic Acid Peel in Treatment of Acne: A Randomized Open-label Study

Rathod D, Pandya P, Pandya I, et al. Comparison of efficacy of commercially available versus freshly prepared salicylic acid peel in treatment of acne: a randomized open-label study.
Biomed Dermatol. 2018;2(1):25.

Abstract

Chemical peels are used for a variety of skin indications like acne, pigmentation and photoaging. The objective of this study was to compare the efficacy of freshly prepared and commercially available salicylic acid (SA) peels in acne. This was a prospective, randomized, open-label, parallel-group study with 126 patients. Subjects were randomized to receive 30% salicylic acid peel either commercially available or freshly prepared. Follow-up and assessment was done every 2 weeks up to 12 weeks. Total acne score was used for objective assessment and subjective assessment was done by visual analog scale. After six sessions with commercially available SA peel, reduction in the average number of comedones was 88.45%, in inflammatory papules 89.16%, in pustules 31.47% and in nodules/cyst 50%. After six sessions with freshly prepared SA peel, reduction in the average number of comedones was 89%, in inflammatory papules 90.36%, pustules 28.3% and in nodules 96%. Significant improvement of both noninflammatory and inflammatory acne was seen in both groups.

COMMENT

Acne is a common disorder of the pilosebaceous glands. Topical and systemic therapies are the mainstay in the management of acne. Novel adjunctive therapies like chemical peels, lasers and photodynamic therapy are on the rise to meet the patient expectations of early cure. Chemical peeling is the application of a chemical agent to the skin that causes controlled destruction of part/whole epidermis with/without dermis leading to exfoliation and removal of superficial lesions followed by rejuvenation of new epidermal and dermal tissues. Salicylic acid (SA) is a hydroxy acid which has been used as a well-tolerated and safe peeling agent in all skin types. It is an excellent keratolytic agent by way of its ability to dissolve intercellular cement thereby reducing corneocytes adhesion. This property of SA accounts for its strong comedolytic effect and its utility in the treatment of acne.

Various preparations of SA are available with huge price differences. This study was carried out to study the safety and efficacy of freshly prepared and commercially available SA peels in acne. This was a prospective, randomized, open-label, parallel-group study with 126 patients. Subjects were randomized to receive 30% SA peel either commercially available or freshly prepared. The peel was applied in a clockwise manner from the forehead. Most patients experienced a stinging sensation during peeling that usually lasted for 3–5 minutes. The end point was development of uniform white crystalline precipitate, "pseudofrost," in the peeled areas. In patients who did not develop the pseudofrost, the cessation of the stinging sensation was considered the end point. As soon as the end point was reached, the peel was neutralized by asking the patients to wash their faces with copious water. Assessment of acne lesions was done at baseline and at 2, 4, 6, 8, 10 and 12 weeks. Both commercially available and freshly prepared SA peels were effective in reducing the number of comedones and papules but less effective in treating nodules and pustules. Noninflammatory and inflammatory lesions were seen to clear faster than would ordinarily have occurred with traditional therapy. There was no difference in the efficacy of freshly prepared versus commercially available SA.

Key Message
- Both freshly prepared and commercially available SA led to a highly significant improvement in the total acne score; freshly prepared SA peel showed improvement significantly earlier at 6 weeks onward.

ARTICLE 43

A Comparison of Combined Oral Contraceptives Containing Chlormadinone Acetate versus Drospirenone for the Treatment of Acne and Dysmenorrhea: A Randomized Trial

Jaisamrarn U, Santibenchakul S. A comparison of combined oral contraceptives containing chlormadinone acetate versus drospirenone for the treatment of acne and dysmenorrhea: a randomized trial. *Contracep Reprod Med. 2018;3(1):5.*

Abstract

Oral contraceptives (OCs) have been used for various other indications other than contraception. Acne is one of the common indications. In this study, comparison was done between the efficacy of OCs containing ethinyl estradiol (EE) and chlormadinone acetate (CMA) versus OCs containing EE and drospirenone (DRSP) for the treatment of acne and dysmenorrhea. It was an investigator-blinded, randomized, parallel-group study conducted in women aged between 18 years and 45 years. About 180 subjects were randomly assigned into two treatment groups, either EE/CMA at the dosage of 30 mcg/2 mg once daily (OD) or EE/DRSP at the dosage of 30 mcg/3 mg OD and evaluated for efficacy for the treatment of acne and dysmenorrhea at baseline visit and after 1, 3 and 6 months of treatment. At 6 months, there was a significant reduction of total acne lesion in the EE/CMA group than EE/DRSP. On grading with the investigator's global assessment of acne treatment, the proportion of the subjects from the EE/CMA group that were rated "excellent" was higher than those from the EE/DRSP. Subjects from the EE/CMA group graded their improvement in acne as "excellent" compared to the EE/DRSP group. EE/CMA group subjects reported a much decrease or absence in dysmenorrheic pain as early as 1 month. The treatments were generally well-tolerated in both groups. There were no significant differences between both groups for adverse events.

COMMENT

Oral contraceptives (OCs) other than having high contraceptive efficacy and safety profile, also have noncontraceptive benefits such as for the skin, hair and menstrual cycle-related disorders. Newer contraceptives have lesser content of ethinyl estradiol (EE), which has resulted in reduced side effects. Progestogens contribute to the distinctive and unique noncontraceptive benefit of OC. The estrogen component of EE remains the same among different combined OCs, the progestogen component varies according to the different brands. Progestogens with weak or no androgenic effects or mild antiandrogen effects are preferred in the management of acne. Chlormadinone acetate (CMA) and drospirenone (DRSP) are the commonly used progestogens.

The EE/CMA is a monophasic combined low-dose OC containing CMA 2.0 mg and EE 30 mcg per tablet, this progestogen has mild antiandrogen effect. EE/DRSP is a monophasic combined OC containing DRSP 3.0 mg and EE 30 mcg per tablet. Drospirenone has antiandrogenic and antimineralocorticoid effects but has negligible estrogenic or glucocorticoid activity. In this study, the authors have compared the efficacy of EE/CMA and EE/DRSP for the treatment of acne and dysmenorrhea among women aged between 18 years and 45 years in a randomized controlled trial.

The study was conducted from August 2013 to October 2017 at the Family Planning Clinic, Department of Obstetrics and Gynaecology, Faculty of Medicine, Chulalongkorn University, Bangkok, Thailand.

There were no significant differences in treatment compliance among the two groups. There were no significant differences in the number of comedones, papules, pustules/nodules and total acne lesions at baseline between the EE/CMA group and EE/DRSP group. Both the drugs were effective in reducing the acne lesions during the 6 months. The EE/CMA group showed significantly more reduction in the acne count, especially the comedones and papules. As per the investigator's global assessment of acne treatment efficacy 75.3% of the subjects in the EE/CMA group, were rated as having an "excellent" response in comparison to 49.4% in the EE/DRSP group. Even in the subjects' self-assessment for acne treatment efficacy, 63.3% of the subjects in the EE/CMA rated the treatment as "excellent" while 48.3% of the subjects in the EE/DRSP rated the treatment as "excellent".

Both treatments were well-tolerated by both the groups and there was no significant difference in side effects. No significant changes in weight were noted.

Key Message
- The EE/CMA is more effective for the treatment of acne and dysmenorrhea in women with mild-to-moderate acne vulgaris and dysmenorrhea than EE/DRSP.

ARTICLE 44

Efficacy and Adverse Events of Oral Isotretinoin for Acne: A Systematic Review

Vallerand IA, Lewinson RT, Farris MS, et al. Efficacy and adverse events of oral isotretinoin for acne: a systematic review. *Brit J Dermatol. 2018;178(1):76-85.*

Abstract

Oral isotretinoin is considered as the gold standard in the management of severe acne. This review is about the efficacy and adverse effects of isotretinoin for acne from 11 different trials. Majority of patients were males, with age ranging from 18 years to 47.9 years. Isotretinoin was found to be more effective than antibiotics or placebo across all trials. Across trials with an overall low risk of bias, two-thirds demonstrated statistically significant differences between isotretinoin and control. The frequency of adverse events was twice as high with isotretinoin (n = 751 events) compared to control (n = 388 events). More than half of all adverse events were dermatologic and related to dryness. Adverse events from isotretinoin causing participant withdrawal from trials (n = 12 patients) included Stevens-Johnson syndrome, cheilitis, xerosis, acne flare, photophobia, elevated liver enzymes, decreased appetite, headaches and depressed mood.

COMMENT

Acne vulgaris is a common skin disorder with adolescence, associated with scarring, postinflammatory hyperpigmentation, psychological distress in the form of anxiety, reduced self-esteem and depression. Isotretinoin is used extensively in the management of moderate-to-severe acne. In this review, the authors have summarized the results of various randomized clinical trials for acne to compare its clinical efficacy and adverse effects with placebo or alternate therapies.

All the trials reported clinically significant reductions in lesion counts with isotretinoin compared to controls and placebo. Compared to antibiotics like minocycline, tetracycline, dapsone, doxycycline, erythromycin and azithromycin isotretinoin reduced acne severity more.

The frequency of adverse events was about twice as high in the isotretinoin groups compared to controls. Approximately two adverse events occurred per patient receiving isotretinoin and approximately one adverse event occurred per control patient. About 3.2% of patients withdrew from the isotretinoin group and 1.8% from the control group due to adverse effects. Cheilitis and xerosis were the most common clinical side effects. Other side effects noted were acne flare and photophobia. One patient had Stevens-Johnson syndrome. Reports of abnormal blood work were more frequent among isotretinoin groups compared to control but the overall frequency of a blood work abnormality was low for both isotretinoin and control. Elevated serum lipids or liver enzymes were the most common biochemical alterations. Gastrointestinal side effects were much lesser compared to antibiotics group. Nausea and vomiting were more frequent with antibiotic therapy (doxycycline and minocycline) compared to isotretinoin. Ocular and ENT side effects were noted more frequently due to the drying effect on the mucosa. However, it was not severe to cause any patients withdrawal from the trial. Psychiatric side effects were reported more frequently in the isotretinoin group compared to controls (0.5%) patients in the isotretinoin group withdrew from the study due to psychiatric symptoms such as depressed mood, insomnia and hallucinations.

Key Message
- Isotretinoin is superior to systemic antibiotics and placebo in reducing acne, and is associated with side effects which are mostly mild. The incidence of serious adverse effects is less.

ARTICLE 45

Aromatherapy, Botanicals, and Essential Oils in Acne

Winkelman WJ. Aromatherapy, botanicals, and essential oils in acne.
Clin Dermatol. 2018;36(3):299-305.

Abstract

Complementary and alternative medicine approaches are well-accepted among some patient populations due to the perception that they are "naturally available" and thus are less likely to be dangerous and these are considered as safe and free of side effects. These include aromatherapy, botanicals, and essential oils (plant extracts). Preliminary evidence suggests these may have some effect on acne especially the biological activity studies, and small pilot clinical trials conducted outside of North America suggest it. When additional research and larger clinical trials are conducted, both clinicians and patients will be able to understand the risks/benefits compared with allopathic remedies.

COMMENT

Complementary and alternative medicine (CAM) is popular among various sections of patients. It is perceived to be more natural, and thus less toxic and safe compared to allopathic medicines. Patients seek CAM in chronic conditions, and acne is one such condition. In this review, essential oils and aromatherapy on acne are evaluated. Botanicals refer to plant-based molecules. Essential oils are botanicals that are volatile plant extracts with distinctive scents and are mixed in a gel, compounded into a paste or spray, or applied via bath, massage, or inhalation. These oils are believed to be absorbed through the upper dermis. Aromatherapy refers to the therapeutic use of aromatic essential oils.

Tea tree oils contain approximately 100 terpenes and are known to have anti-inflammatory action. There are several studies with tea tree oil in acne and their efficacy is found to be similar to benzoyl peroxide with lesser side effects, however, the onset of action is slower. *Lactobacillus* Fermented *Chamaecyparis obtusa* (LFCO) leaf extract has strong inhibitory effects on *Propionibacterium acnes*. In comparison to tea tree oil, LFCO has a faster onset of action and a greater effect on inflammation and inflammatory markers. LFCO is also sebosuppressive and associated with a reduction in the size of sebaceous glands, with concomitant lower sebum output. *Copaiba* is an oil-resin, the therapeutic actions primarily attributed to diterpene compounds. In comparison to placebo, copaiba oil has shown to reduce the number of inflammatory acne lesions. Sandalwood oil has antibacterial actions against *Staphylococcus aureus, Staphylococcus epidermidis*, and *P. acnes* at concentrations of 0.06% and lower. Anti-inflammatory effects are thought to occur via inhibition of COX-1 and COX-2, and 12-lipoxygenase pathways. Sandalwood oil 0.5% formulated with salicylic acid for acne showed 89% improvement in patients in reduction of acne as well as spots. Rosemary extract contains three bioactive compounds: rosmarinic acid, carnosol and carnosic acid. Addition of rosemary extract contributes to anti-inflammatory actions to cosmeceutical or dermatologic products. Jeju essential oil is derived from *Thymus* plants and is said to have antibacterial effect against *P. acnes*.

Key Message

- There is a weak clinical evidence for the use of CAM in acne. Many of these agents may be used as complementary therapy in the management of their acne.

ARTICLE 46

A Review of Diagnosis and Treatment of Acne in Adult Female Patients

Tan AU, Schlosser BJ, Paller AS. A review of diagnosis and treatment of acne in adult female patients. *Int J Women's Dermatol.* 2018;4(2):56-71.

Abstract

Acne in women may start during adolescence and continue beyond the age of 25 years, or it may have its onset after the age of 25 years. The objective of this review was to evaluate the treatment options in adult female patients with acne. Management of adult acne is associated with various challenges such as pregnancy, lactation, and hormonal disturbances. Treatment is planned according to each patient's severity, associated symptoms and preferences. This study reviews the conventional therapies, alternative therapies, and newer modalities in the management of adult acne.

COMMENT

Acne is a very common condition of the pilosebaceous unit, with a prevalence of about 85% in adolescents, 50.9% in ages of 20-29 years and 26.3% in women of 40-49 years. The pathogenesis of acne in adult females is quite complex. Androgens play a major role here, evidenced by the presence of acne in hyperandrogenic conditions such as PCOS and response of acne to hormonal therapy. Androgens stimulate sebum production via androgen receptors on the sebaceous glands. Distribution of acne on the lower half of the face suggests it to be hormonal distribution. Persistent acne, which is acne that persists beyond adolescence into adulthood, is the most common type of acne in adult women.

While evaluating an adult woman with acne menstrual history and examination for signs of hyperandrogenism such as hirsutism, seborrhea, androgenetic alopecia, virilization, etc. should be looked for. When there is a failure of multiple courses of antibiotic therapy and isotretinoin therapy, hormonal acne should be investigated for.

Commonly used topical treatments for patients with acne include benzoyl peroxide (BP), salicylic acid (SA), antibiotic medications, combination antibiotic medications with BP, retinoid medications, retinoid with BP, retinoid with antibiotic medication, azelaic acid, and sulfone agents. Among systemic therapy, tetracycline group of antibiotics, which include minocycline, doxycycline, and tetracycline, are considered among the first-line therapy in patients with moderate-to-severe inflammatory acne. Trimethoprim-sulfamethoxazole (TMP/SMX) can be used to treat patients with AV that is recalcitrant to macrolide and tetracycline. Isotretinoin is an important non-hormonal and non-antimicrobial treatment option for adult women with acne, isotretinoin is usually initiated at a starting dose of 0.5 mg/kg/day for the first month and then increased to 1 mg/kg/day as tolerated with a goal of a cumulative dose of between 120 mg/kg and 150 mg/kg. In the treatment of adult women, serious considerations should be given to isotretinoin's potential teratogenicity.

Miscellaneous therapies which are used as adjuvants to oral and systemic therapy are comedo extraction, cryotherapy, electrocauterization, chemical peels, and microdermabrasion.

In this study, the hormonal therapy for acne is not reviewed which forms the mainstay of therapy in adult acne.

Key Messages

- While treating adult acne factors such as pregnancy and lactation should be considered
- Evaluation for signs for hyperandrogenism to be done when there is a failure to isotretinoin therapy or relapse soon after.

ARTICLE 47

Clinical Evidence for Washing and Cleansers in Acne Vulgaris: A Systematic Review

Stringer T, Nagler A, Orlow SJ, et al. Clinical evidence for washing and cleansers in acne vulgaris: a systematic review. J Dermatol Treat. 2018;29(7):688-93.

Abstract

Along with topical and systemic medications, face washes and cleansers are also used commonly for acne. They may either be prescribed by physician or patients procure it over the counter. The clinical benefit of these washes and cleansers is poorly established. The objective of this study was to review the clinical studies of washing and cleanser efficacy in acne vulgaris and to guide treatment recommendations for dermatologists. Fourteen prospective studies were surveyed. Modalities investigated included face washing frequency, true soap/syndet cleansing bars, antiseptic cleansers, alpha and beta-hydroxy (i.e. salicylic) acid cleansers, and several proprietary formulations. Given the low number of well-performed clinical studies of cleansers and washing, it is difficult to formulate reliable recommendations.

COMMENT

Acne is a common chronic condition. Patients perceive acne to be due to poor skin hygiene and often use face washes and cleansers before consulting dermatologists. None of the standard recommendations and guidelines for acne comment about cleansers or face washes. The relative absence of studies combined with the multitude of available agents makes appropriate product selection challenging for practitioners and patients alike. In this review, the authors have included prospective studies in which the impact of washing frequency or non-prescription cleansers on acne vulgaris was included.

A single-blinded randomized controlled trial for the frequency of face washes showed that there was a significant increase in the acne count in those who washed once a day, significantly lower count in those who washed twice daily and no change in those who washed four times a day.

Soaps are of three types, true soaps—comprised of an alkali and a fatty acid, syndet which use synthetic surfactants, and combars, which include features of both. Syndet bars are found to be superior to soaps in reducing inflammatory lesions. Gentle liquid skin cleansers are agents which use surface-active emulsifiers to remove dirt, sebum, bacteria and corneocytes. Studies comparing cleansing gels with skin creams have shown significant reduction in acne count with cleansing gels. A chlorhexidine gluconate cleanser has shown to reduce the mean comedone count, but there are often reported incidences of skin irritation. Benzoyl peroxide foam issued commonly for truncal acne. The short contact time has shown a significant reduction in *Propionibacterium acnes* colony count. Various studies on combination therapy of benzoyl peroxide cleansers with topical tretinoin have shown a significant reduction in acne counts. Face washes using glycolic acid and salicylic acid are used extensively. There are reports of their efficacy in reducing acne. However, their effectiveness as monotherapy in acne is yet to be determined.

Key Message

- *The amount of clinical data available about efficacy of cleansers and washes in acne is not sufficient enough to have them included in the acne management guidelines.*

ARTICLE 48

ROS-responsive Microneedle Patch for Acne Vulgaris Treatment

Zhang Y, Feng P, Yu J, et al. ROS-responsive microneedle patch for acne vulgaris treatment.
Adv Therap. 2018;1(3):01-06.

Abstract

Acne vulgaris is a common inflammatory disorder of pilosebaceous glands associated with colonization of *Propionibacterium acnes* (*P. acnes*). Though topical therapies like antibiotics are prescribed routinely, the delivery of these drugs within the pilosebaceous glands is less, leading to poor bactericidal effect. Here, the authors have described a new method of drug administration using a reactive oxygen species (ROS)-responsive microneedle (MN) patch. In response to the over-generated ROS within acne, it is important to have a controlled and sustained drug release. This also aids in improving the antibacterial effect and reducing the side effects. The patch base, formed by hyaluronic acid (HA) and diatomaceous earth (DE) with high physical adsorption capability, accelerates healing of skin through the absorption of pus and dead cell debris. Studies in *P. acnes*-induced mouse model has demonstrated this bioresponsive patch with adsorption capability, could efficiently reduce the skin swelling and inhibit the bacterial growth.

COMMENT

Acne vulgaris is a chronic inflammatory disorder of pilosebaceous gland with a prevalence of about 85% among adolescents. Blockage of the pilosebaceous duct, proliferation of *P. acnes* in the duct, and hyperkeratinization of the duct are the factors in the pathogenesis of acne. *Propionibacterium acnes* is a gram-positive anaerobic bacterium that has a crucial role in the development of inflammatory acne. The lipases in *P. acnes* catalyzes the hydrolysis of sebum triglycerides to free fatty acids, which disrupts the follicular epithelium. The chemotactic factors secreted by *P. acnes*, results in accumulation of inflammatory cells and mediators which exacerbated the inflammation. Commonly used topical antibiotics are erythromycin and clindamycin. These agents have poor penetration up to the dermis, and may not be very effective in targeting *P. acnes*.

Here, the authors have used microneedles (MNs) to enhance the penetration of antibiotics. MNs was prepared from a drug-loaded reactive oxygen species (ROS)-responsive poly(vinyl alcohol) (RR-PVA) matrix. ROS-responsive MNs were able to release drug within the *P. acnes*-infected follicle in a sustained manner once penetrating through epidermis, thus enabled effective inhibition of the proliferation of bacteria. A methacrylated hyaluronic acid (m-HA)/diatomaceous earth (DE) contained base was utilized as the supporting substrate for MNs, which may adsorb pus as well as other purulent exudates and debris for promoted healing. A transparent plastic film was further applied to cover the patch as a waterproof, sterile barrier to external contaminants. The in vivo antibacterial performance of MN patches was investigated in a *P. acnes*-induced inflammation mouse model. The investigative group of mice showed significant reduction in skin swelling, suggesting the effective inhibitory effect of MN patch on acne growth.

Key Message

- ROS-responsive microneedle patch seems like a promising drug delivery technique to deliver the drugs up to the dermis and pilosebaceous units.

ARTICLE 49

Optimizing the Use of Topical Retinoids in Asian Acne Patients

See JA, Goh CL, Hayashi N, et al. Optimizing the use of topical retinoids in Asian acne patients.
J Dermatol. 2018;45(5):522-8.

Abstract

Acne vulgaris is a common disorder across all races. Topical retinoids are the standard agents in topical therapy. They are underutilized in Asian populations probably due to the perception that Asian skin has an increased tendency of sensitivity compared to Caucasians. In this review, the authors have discussed the use of topical retinoids among Asians.

COMMENT

Acne is a common disorder of the pilosebaceous glands with a prevalence of about 80% during adolescence. Fitzpatrick skin type IV to VI have a higher incidence of scarring and postinflammatory pigmentation post acne. Both postinflammatory pigmentation and scarring cause a psychological impact on the patients. Some studies have shown that the tolerability to retinoids is lesser among these skin types. Climate in the Asian countries is tropical which may also have a bearing on tolerability of retinoids. Topical retinoids, antibiotics, and benzoyl peroxide are the commonly used medications for mild-to-moderate acne. Topical retinoids have replaced antibiotics as the first-line choice of topical therapy. Retinoids not only reduce the comedones, they also have effect on the inflammatory lesions of acne. So, they are ideal for clearing lesions and also for maintenance, as they reduce the microcomedones which are precursors for inflammatory acne lesions.

Topical retinoids result in skin sensitivity like dryness and erythema. This can be managed by prescribing a good moisturizer and a cleansing lotion, advising the patient to use sunscreens, avoid too much sun exposure. The retinoid may be used on alternate days or for a shorter period of time during the first 2 weeks to let the skin adaptation occur. Other advantage of using retinoids is its effect in reducing postinflammatory pigmentation. Patient compliance and adherence to treatment can be improved by proper counseling and modifying the regimens. Studies comparing the combination of clindamycin and benzoyl peroxide with retinoids have shown that the tolerability to both the agents is similar among Asians. Though the efficacy of adapalene and tretinoin were the same in reducing the number of acne lesions, skin irritation was experienced more with tretinoin.

Key Message

- Topical retinoids are the first choice among topical therapy for acne as they reduce comedones, inflammatory lesions as well as pigmentation.

ARTICLE 50

Comparative Study of the Efficacy of Platelet-rich Plasma Combined with Carboxytherapy versus its Use with Fractional Carbon Dioxide Laser in Atrophic Acne Scars

Al Taweel AI, Al Refae AA, Hamed AM, et al. Comparative study of the efficacy of Platelet-rich plasma combined with carboxytherapy vs. its use with fractional carbon dioxide laser in atrophic acne scars.
J Cosmet Dermatol. 2019;18(1):150-5.

Abstract

Acne scar is a cause for major psychological morbidity in individuals. Treatment of acne scars is mainly nonpharmacological. Platelet-rich plasma (PRP) and fractional CO_2 lasers are innovative treatment modalities for acne scars. Carboxytherapy can also be used to improve scar tissue through the increase in collagen deposition and reorganization, and the improvement in skin texture and tone. The objective of this study was to compare the efficacy, safety, and complications of the intradermal injection of PRP combined with carboxytherapy and PRP combined with fractional CO_2 laser, in the treatment of atrophic acne scars. Twenty patients were treated with each of the above therapies and the results evaluated. Though the combination of fractional CO_2 with PRP showed better results, side effects were also more.

COMMENT

Acne scar is an unfortunate sequel of acne and may result in poor self-esteem, depression, anxiety, impaired social interactions, body image alterations, embarrassment, anger, lowered academic performance, and unemployment. Many treatments are available for acne scar, and most of them are nonpharmacological like chemical peels, lasers, dermabrasion, fillers and surgery. Even with all the treatment, there will not be 100% clearance of acne scars. For optimal results combination treatment is always preferred.

Platelet-rich plasma treatment is performed via the autologous injection of a high concentration of platelets in a small volume of plasma. It is used increasingly in the management of ulcers, androgenetic alopecia, and as fillers for atrophic scars. There are more than 30 bioactive substances in these granules such as platelet-derived growth factor (PDGF), transforming growth factor (TGF)-β1, 2, epidermal growth factor, and mitogenic growth factors such as platelet-derived angiogenesis factor and fibrinogen.

Fractional ablative carbon dioxide (CO_2) laser (FCL) therapy is based on the theory of fractional photothermolysis creating microscopic channels of thermal injury in the skin. Reepithelization results in skin tightening and smoothening; collagen remodeling improves depressed scars.

Carboxytherapy refers to the cutaneous and subcutaneous administration of CO_2 for therapeutic purposes. The tissue stretching during infusion induces a sub-clinical inflammation, which triggers tissue regeneration processes that induce the activation of macrophages, fibroblasts, and endothelial cells that stimulate remodeling of the extracellular matrix. This improves blood flow, vascularization, collagen synthesis, skin elasticity, appearance of fine lines and wrinkles, and destroys localized fatty deposits. It is more economical and safe also.

In this study, 20 patients were subjected to three sessions of PRP intradermal injection after fractional CO_2 laser with 1 month apart (group A). The other 20 patients were subjected to three sessions of PRP intradermal injection, and then, CO_2 gas was injected intradermally in the area of scars using a 30G needle with flow 80 cc/min (group B). The clinical endpoint of each injection was at the occurrence of an erythema and distension of the injected tissue. Evaluation of patients' improvement indicated a statistically significant improvement of acne scars in group A compared to group B, with no statistically significant differences between the two groups in patients' satisfaction. Side effects like pain during the procedure, edema and erythema post procedure were significantly more with group A. PRP after laser procedure helps in faster recovery of laser damaged skin and also synergistically improves clinical appearance of acne scars.

Key Message

- Improvement of acne scars was noted in both treatment modalities with statistically significant results in favor of fractional CO_2 laser but with more side effects. Carboxytherapy is a promising tool in treatment of acne scars with less complication.

ARTICLE 51

Effects of Oral Supplementation with FOS and GOS Prebiotics in Women with Adult Acne: The "SO Sweet" Study: A Proof-of-concept Pilot Trial

Dall'Oglio F, Milani M, Micali G. Effects of oral supplementation with FOS and GOS prebiotics in women with adult acne: the "SO Sweet" study: a proof-of-concept pilot trial.
Clin Cosmet Investig Dermatol. 2018;11:445.

Abstract

In this study, the authors have evaluated the effects of 3-month prebiotic oral supplementation with fructooligosaccharides (FOS) and galactooligosaccharides (GOS) on glucose and lipid metabolic parameters in 12 adult women with acne. Subjects were treated with a food supplement containing FOS (100 mg) and GOS (500 mg), one sachet daily, for 3 months. Levels of fasting blood glucose, blood insulin, glycated hemoglobin, C peptide, triglycerides, and total cholesterol were evaluated at baseline baseline visit (T0), at month 1 (T1), and at month 3 (T2). No modification in BMI was observed during the study. A significant reduction was observed in fasting glucose levels, total cholesterol, and triglycerides levels. Insulin and C-peptide plasma levels showed a non-significant reduction trend from baseline to the end of the study. This study showed that supplementation with prebiotic FOS and GOS was associated with positive effects on glycemic and lipid metabolic parameters.

COMMENT

Acne which persists after the age of 25 or onset of acne in women over the age of 25 years is called adult acne. Adult acne is associated with genetic factors, hyperandrogenism, metabolic syndrome, and high glycemic index. Few studies have shown elevated insulin levels in an adult female with acne. Chronic and acute hyperinsulinemia upregulates the production of insulin-like growth factor-1 (IGF-1), which is a potent mitogen stimulating cellular growth at the follicle level. Both insulin and IGF-1 stimulate the production of androgens in ovarian and testicular tissues. In obese subjects, therapeutic modification of intestinal microbiota is associated with an improvement of insulin sensitivity. Fructooligosaccharides (FOS) and galactooligosaccharides (GOS) are prebiotic substances able to improve intestinal microbiota. Experimental data show that oral supplementation with FOS and GOS could have a positive effect on glucose metabolism in healthy nondiabetic individuals, thereby reducing the glycemic diet load effects. This study was designed to study the effects of prebiotic oral supplementation with FOS and GOS on glucose and lipid metabolic parameters in women with adult acne.

Twelve adult women with acne were included in the study. Subjects were treated with a food supplement containing FOS (100 mg) and GOS (500 mg), one sachet daily, for 3 months. Levels of fasting blood glucose, blood insulin glycated hemoglobin, C peptide, triglycerides, and total cholesterol were evaluated at baseline visit (T0), at month 1 (T1), and at month 3 (T2). No modification in BMI was observed during the study. A significant reduction was observed in fasting glucose levels, total cholesterol, and triglycerides levels. Insulin and C-peptide plasma levels showed a non-significant reduction trend from baseline to the end of the study.

The normal microbial biofilm is manly contributed by *Bifidobacterium*, loss of this biofilm occurs in high sugar and fat diets. Oral nutritional supplementation with prebiotics like FOS and GOS has been demonstrated to increase stool colony counts of *Bifidobacterium* and Lactobacilli, contributing to maintain efficient intestinal mucosal barrier. Prebiotics could improve insulin sensitivity, thus, controlling the role of high glycemic diets in acne exacerbation.

Key Message

- *Oral supplementation with prebiotic FOS and GOS was associated with positive effects on glycemic and lipid metabolism parameters. Their exact effect on adult acne has to be evaluated further.*

ARTICLE 52

Approaches to Limit Systemic Antibiotic Use in Acne: Systemic Alternatives, Emerging Topical Therapies, Dietary Modification, and Laser and Light-based Treatments

Barbieri JS, Spaccarelli N, Margolis DJ, et al. Approaches to limit systemic antibiotic use in acne: Systemic alternatives, emerging topical therapies, dietary modification, and laser and light-based treatments.
J Am Acad Dermatol. 2019;80(2):538-49.

Abstract

Oral antibiotics are the most commonly used systemic therapy for acne. Extensive use of oral antibiotics is associated with unwanted outcomes like resistance and disruption of microbiome. Though various guidelines in acne management do not advocate antibiotics as the first line of therapy, the scenario in clinical practice is otherwise. In this review article, the authors have compiled the available alternate therapies for acne including the various topical and systemic therapies, laser- and light-based devices.

COMMENT

Acne is a common chronic condition. Antibiotics are one of the extensively prescribed medications for acne especially the tetracycline group. Increased reports of resistance of *Cutibacterium* to acne are known. Other than the development of resistance, antibiotics are also associated with disruption of the normal flora, bacterial resistance among other organisms, and increased rates of upper respiratory infection. Though acne guidelines do not recommend antibiotics as the first line of therapy, in clinical practice antibiotics are prescribed extensively for acne. This article has reviewed the available alternate options.

Due to the effect on sebum production through inhibition of the androgen receptor on sebocytes, spironolactone is a good alternative for antibiotics. Its use should not be limited only to adult women or women with prominent acne on the lower face or acne that flares with their menstrual flares. Menstrual irregularities are the most common complication noted which is usually dose dependent. Oral contraceptives containing estrogen and progestin reduce free testosterone by 40-50% on average. The drospirenone containing oral contraceptives are preferred. A course of 3-6 months of therapy is typically required for patients to experience the full benefit of treatment with combined oral contraceptives (COC).

Isotretinoin is typically started at 0.5 mg/kg/day and uptitrated to 1 mg/kg/day as tolerated. There is evidence that higher cumulative doses of isotretinoin are associated with decreased rates of relapse. Isotretinoin is the only acne medication that alters the course of the disease with effect on all the pathogenetic mechanisms of acne.

Topical retinoids, benzoyl peroxide, and topical antibiotics have been a mainstay of the topical management of acne for decades. Topical medications aiming to suppress sebum production are an emerging approach. Enzyme stearoyl-coenzyme A desaturase 1 (SCD1) is a potential target for reducing sebum production. Several clinical trials of topical formulations of SCD1 are ongoing. Nitric oxide-releasing particles are under investigation due to their potential to suppress the release of multiple cytokines from human monocytes and keratinocytes and to prevent *C. acnes*-induced inflammation. In a recent randomized trial evaluating 46 patients treated with either 5-aminolevulinic acid (5-ALA) photodynamic therapy (PDT) followed by adapalene 0.1% gel or oral doxycycline 100 mg/day plus adapalene gel, a greater reduction of inflammatory and total lesion counts was found in PDT group in 12 weeks. IPL has been explored due to its potential to destroy C. acnes and induce thermolysis of blood vessels supplying the sebaceous glands, thereby reducing sebum production. To improve efficacy and reduce side effects of laser-based treatments, attempts have been made to concentrate the thermal injury to the sebaceous glands while sparing surrounding structures using gold-coated silica and silver microparticles.

Milk consumption has been suggested to play a potential role in the pathogenesis of acne by increasing insulin and IGF-1 levels. Results from several retrospective and prospective observational studies have suggested a potential association between milk consumption and acne.

Key Message

- Emerging topical therapies, laser- and light-based modalities, dietary modification, spironolactone, COCs, and isotretinoin can all be effective therapeutic alternatives in the appropriate clinical context for acne.

ARTICLE 53

The Efficacy and Tolerability of 5-aminolevulinic Acid 5% Thermosetting Gel Photodynamic Therapy in the Treatment of Mild-to-moderate Acne Vulgaris. A Two-center, Prospective Assessor-blinded, Proof-of-concept Study

Serini SM, Cannizzaro MV, Dattola A, et al. The efficacy and tolerability of 5-aminolevulinic acid 5% thermosetting gel photodynamic therapy (PDT) in the treatment of mild-to-moderate acne vulgaris. A two-center, prospective assessor-blinded, proof-of-concept study.
J Cosmet Dermatol. 2019;18(1):156-62.

Abstract

Acne is a chronic inflammatory condition with a high prevalence. Though topical antibiotics, retinoids, and benzoyl peroxide are the cornerstones in the management, search is continuously on for new formulations and molecules which will provide better adherence and lower resistance. Photodynamic therapy (PDT) with 20% aminolevulinic acid (ALA) has shown to be effective in the treatment of inflammatory acne. Skin tolerability was an issue with this. This study was designed to study the efficacy and tolerability of 630 nm PDT with a new 5-ALA "low-dose" topical gel formulation (5%) in the treatment of inflammatory mild-to-moderate acne vulgaris (AV). This new gel formulation allows convenient application without occlusion and a more efficient release of active particles compared to traditional ALA formulations. Thirty-five patients with mild-to-moderate acne were enrolled in the study. Global Acne Grade System (GAG) score was performed at baseline and after an average of three, 630-nm, 15-minute PDT sessions, performed every 2 weeks. GAG score was also calculated in a follow-up visit 6 months after the last PDT session. Significant reduction in the score was noticed at the end of the study and the drug was also well tolerated.

COMMENT

Acne is a common chronic disorder. As with any other chronic diseases, adherence to therapy is the major hindrance in delivering effective treatment. The principle of photodynamic therapy (PDT) is that specific wavelengths of light irradiation combined with local or systemic use of photosensitizer generate oxygen and free radicals. Blue-light (405 nm) and red-light (630 nm) lamps are commonly used. PDT involves the application of a photosensitizing chemical, 5-aminolevulinic acid (5-ALA) which, when exposed to various lights, results in excitation of the photosensitizer [protoporphyrin IX (PpIX)] and the consequent production of a reactive oxygen species that leads to cytotoxicity. Blue light (405 nm) is the most potent wavelength for activation of endogenous PpIX components of *Propionibacterium acnes*. However, blue light has a poor depth penetration into the skin (about 1 mm). In contrast, red light (635 nm) can penetrate deeper (about 3 mm). Red-light PDT is considered very effective in inducing inhibition and destruction of sebaceous gland. Skin tolerability is an issue with PDT. To overcome this a low dose 5% ALA was developed. This low-dose ALA allows a more convenient application procedure without occlusion and better and more efficient release of the active compound in comparison with traditional ALA formulations like creams or ointments. This gel contains a peculiar polymer, poloxamer 407, which is liquid at room temperature and becomes a semi-solid (gel) when in contact with the skin. The advantage of this thermosetting gel is that occlusion is not required. The application of the gel without occlusion facilitates the use and improved the patients' compliance. The clinical results were comparable to 20% ALA with reduced side effects and better skin tolerability.

Key Message

- This is a therapeutic option in moderate-to-severe acne patients in whom isotretinoin is contra-indicated. The low (i.e. 5%) concentration of ALA formulation used in this trial in comparison with traditional "high-concentration" ALA formulations (i.e. 20%) could improve the skin tolerability without losing clinical efficacy.

ARTICLE 54

Combination Chemical Peels are More Effective than Single Chemical Peel in Treatment of Mild-to-moderate Acne Vulgaris: A Split Face Comparative Clinical Trial

Nofal E, Nofal A, Gharib K, et al. Combination chemical peels are more effective than single chemical peel in treatment of mild-to-moderate acne vulgaris: A split face comparative clinical trial.
J Cosmet Dermatol. 2018;00:1-9.

Abstract

Acne is a common problem with profound psychological impact. Treatment of acne is always tailor made and involves choosing the right medication according to the type of acne—mild, moderate, or severe. Chemical peeling is a well-known option in the management of acne vulgaris. This study was done to evaluate and compare clinical efficacy and safety of combination chemical peels versus single peel in the treatment of mild-to-moderate acne. The study included 3 groups of 15 patients each having mild-to-moderate acne. One group was treated with combination sequential peels with modified Jessner's solution (MJ) followed by trichloroacetic acid (TCA 20%) on the right (Rt) side of the face versus TCA 30% on the left (Lt) side. The second group was treated by combination peels of salicylic (20%) mandelic (10%) (SM) mixture on the Rt half versus salicylic acid 30% on the Lt half. The third group underwent combination sequential peeling of MJ and TCA on the Rt side versus SM combination peels on the Lt side. All patients underwent six sessions with 2-week apart and followed up for 3 months after the last session. In all the three groups, the combination peels proved to be more efficacious than the single peel treatments.

COMMENT

This study was a split-face comparative study to evaluate the safety and effectiveness of combination peels in comparison to single peel in patients with mild-to-moderate acne. Chemical peeling is a common modality of treatment in acne. Many chemical agents are utilized to control acne and many factors govern in choosing a particular agent. These agents can be a single agent with various concentrations or a combination of agents. Commonly used agents are 20–30% salicylic acid, 20–70% glycolic acid, 10–30% trichloroacetic acid (TCA), Jessner's solution, Monheit's combination (Jessner's + 35% TCA), Coleman's combination (glycolic 70% + TCA 35%), Barker-Gordon formula (phenol 88% + tap water + liquid soap + croton oil).

This study included 45 patients with mild-to-moderate acne vulgaris who were assigned to three groups. A prepeel test was performed by application of the peeling agent on a 1 cm × 1 cm area in the right retroauricular area. Group A was treated with combination sequential peels of MJ solution followed by TCA 20% in the right side of the face and TCA 30% alone in the left side. In group B, SM was applied on the Rt side of the face whereas plain 30% salicylic acid was applied on the left side. The uniform pseudo frosting was considered end point on both sides. Similarly, In group C, MJ followed by TCA 20% solution was applied on the Rt side of the face and SM was applied on the Lt side. Michaelson acne score and Quartile grading scale and patient satisfaction scale were used in the assessment. Both sides of the face showed significant improvement of acne lesions but improvement was significantly higher and earlier in sides treated by combination peels. Side effects were minimal.

Key Message

- *Combinations of chemical peel are more effective in management of acne than monotherapy.*

ARTICLE 55

Comparison of Efficacy of Aminolevulinic Acid Photodynamic Therapy versus Adapalene Gel plus Oral Doxycycline for Treatment of Moderate Acne Vulgaris – A Simple, Blind, Randomized, and Controlled Trial

Nicklas C, Rubio R, Cárdenas C, et al. Comparison of efficacy of aminolevulinic acid photodynamic therapy versus adapalene gel plus oral doxycycline for treatment of moderate acne vulgaris–a simple, blind, randomized, and controlled trial.
Photodermatol Photoimmunol Photomed. 2019;35(1):3-10.

Abstract

Photodynamic therapy (PDT) using aminolevulinic acid (ALA) is less commonly used treatment option in the management of acne. Also comparative studies with other standard therapies are lacking. This study was a randomized, controlled trial involving 46 patients with moderate inflammatory facial acne, 23 patients received two sessions of PDT separated by 2 weeks (ALA 20% incubated 1.5 hours before red light irradiation with 37 J/cm^2 fluence) and 23 patients received doxycycline 100 mg/day plus adapalene gel 0.1%. At the end of 6 weeks lesional counts were greatly reduced in PDT group than doxycycline plus adapalene. At 12 weeks, there was a greater reduction of inflammatory lesions in PDT group. ALA-PDT offers promise as an alternative treatment for moderately severe inflammatory acne that has a higher effectiveness than the combination of doxycycline and adapalene gel in reducing noninflammatory and total lesions at 6 weeks. There were significantly superior reductions at 12 weeks in the combination of PDT group followed by adapalene gel in total, inflammatory, and noninflammatory lesions.

COMMENT

Acne vulgaris (AV) is a common condition with a global prevalence of 9.4% and affects 15–25 years of age group. It can present as papules, pustules, nodules, cysts, and/or scar. Various treatment modalities are available, but current guidelines recommend topical retinoids along with oral antibiotics for the treatment of moderately severe acne. Long-term antibiotics might lead to resistance in *Propionibacterium acnes*, so alternative therapy like PDT might have advantage. PDT acts as transient antimicrobial, anti-inflammatory agent, and inhibits sebaceous gland and causes long-lasting sebaceous gland destruction. This study is a randomized, controlled, investigator-blinded, and parallel-group trial which compares efficacy of aminolevulinic acid (ALA) photodynamic therapy versus adapalene gel plus oral doxycycline for treatment of moderate AV.

Patients with moderately severe inflammatory AV as per Leeds revised acne grading system with modifications as numerous papules and pustules (40-100) usually with many comedones (40-100) and the occasional (up to 5) larger, deeper nodular inflamed lesions in the face were enrolled. A total of 23 patients were recruited in each study group. Patients in the ALA-PDT group received two treatments session, 2 weeks apart and other group received doxycycline 100 mg/day orally plus adapalene gel 0.1% for 6 weeks. From the sixth week, both groups started adapalene gel 0.1% as maintenance therapy until 12 weeks of follow-up. All patients were evaluated at baseline, at weeks 6 and 12 after the start of treatment by two dermatologists. The median percent reductions in noninflammatory lesion count (p = 0.013) and total lesions (p = 0.038) at 6 weeks was found to be significantly higher in the group receiving PDT. At 12 weeks, there was a greater reduction of inflammatory lesion in PDT group with 84% versus 74% for group who received doxycycline plus adapalene (p = 0.020) as well as in reducing total lesions with 79% versus 67%, respectively (p = 0.026). This study concluded that ALA-PDT with red light offers promise as an alternative treatment for moderately severe inflammatory AV. It had a better effectiveness than the combination of doxycycline and adapalene gel in lowering noninflammatory and total lesional count at the end of 6 weeks of treatment and had a similar effect in reducing the inflammatory lesions. Also, there were significant reductions at the end of 12 weeks in the combination of PDT group followed by adapalene gel relative to the doxycycline and adapalene gel group in total, inflammatory, and noninflammatory lesions. Small sample size and lack of long follow-up are the main limitation factors.

Key Messages
- Photodynamic therapy (PDT) is a potential agent for treatment of acne
- It has antimicrobial, anti-inflammatory, and inhibits sebaceous gland secretion, and causes long-lasting sebaceous gland destruction.

ARTICLE 56

Microneedling by Dermapen and Glycolic Acid Peel for the Treatment of Acne Scars: Comparative Study

Saadawi AN, Esawy AM, Kandeel AH, et al. Microneedling by dermapen and glycolic acid peel for the treatment of acne scars: comparative study.
J Cosmet Dermatol. 2019;18:107-14.

Abstract

Acne scar procedures are associated with high cost and some with low results and complications. The aim of the study was to compare and evaluate the efficacy and safety therapy of 35% glycolic acid (GA) peel, microneedling with dermapen and a combination of both in management of atrophic acne scars. The study included 30 patients suffering from various types of acne scars. Study subjects were randomly assigned into three groups, each group included 10 patients; group I was treated with GA peel, group II treated was with microneedling and group III received a combination of both procedures. Six sessions were done in each group. Qualitative global scar grading system was used to evaluate the clinical assessment before and after treatment, quartile grading scale, and degree of patient satisfaction. Study showed a statistically significant improvement in acne scars grade after treatment among the study groups ($p = 0.04$) but it was higher in group III. Boxcar, ice pick, and rolling scars improved in all groups, respectively ($p = 0.03$, $p = 0.04$, $p = 0.04$). Patients' satisfaction was higher in group III ($p = 0.04$). The study concluded that the combination of dermapen and GA peel is more effective than monotherapy.

COMMENT

Acne scar is challenging to treat and numerous treatments have been described. It includes laser surgery, radiofrequency intervention, chemical peels, chemical reconstruction of skin scars (CROSS) technique, dermabrasion, needling, subcision, punch techniques, fat transplantation, and other tissue augmenting agents. This study evaluates and compares the efficacy and safety of 35% glycolic acid (GA) peel, microneedling with dermapen and a combination of GA 35% peel and micro needling with dermapen in the treatment of acne scars. Three groups of 10 patients were enrolled and response to treatment was assessed using the qualitative global scar grading system before and after treatment, quartile grading scale, and degree of patient satisfaction. Group I, II and III underwent microneedling, GA peel and combination respectively every fortnightly for six sessions. In group III GA peeling and microneedling were done alternately for 3 months. Digital color facial photographs were taken using a digital camera. Left and right profile views were obtained at baseline, before the session, 2 weeks after the last session and at the end of follow-up after 1 month.

Two dermatologists before and after the study, evaluated the photographs and graded as per grading system—very good improvement >75%; good improvement of 50–74%; mild improvement of 25–49%; and poor or no improvement <25%. Degrees of improvement were assessed by participants as no, mild, good, and very good. Pain was assessed by the participants and graded as mild, moderate, and severe. Treatment related side effects such as persistent erythema, post inflammatory hyperpigmentation (PIH), hypopigmentation, herpes simplex flare-up, scarring, or keloids were noted at each session.

The study observed a statistical significant increase in frequency of improvement in rolling compared to boxcar and ice pick in all groups and also in boxcar compared to ice pick in the three groups. Also, study noted statistically significant increase in frequency of "very good" satisfactory and objective variables in group III compared to group I and group II, and in group I compared to group II. The study concluded that combination of dermapen and GA peel is more effective than monotherapy but all the treatments were effective in treating boxcar, ice pick, and rolling scars.

Key Messages
- The study compares two commonly performed procedures for acne scars and also compares combination therapy with isolated procedures
- Rolling scars had better results with therapy
- Combining GA and microneedling is better than single therapy.

ARTICLE 57

Antipruritic Efficacies of Doxycycline and Erythromycin in the Treatment of Acne Vulgaris: A Randomized Single-blinded Pilot Study

Cao T, Tan ET, Chan YH, et al. Antipruritic efficacies of doxycycline and erythromycin in the treatment of acne vulgaris: a randomized single-blinded pilot study.
Ind J Dermatol Venereol Leprol. 2018;84(4):458-60.

Abstract
The objective of this randomized, single-blinded pilot study was to evaluate and compare the antipruritic efficacies of doxycycline and erythromycin in the treatment of acne vulgaris (AV) in 29 subjects. This is a letter to the editor that showed statistically significant reduction in itch intensity scores at 6 weeks with doxycycline and concluded that doxycycline effectively reduces itch intensity in pruritic acne.

COMMENT

This article is a randomized, single-blinded pilot study to evaluate the antipruritic efficacies of doxycycline and erythromycin in the treatment of acne vulgaris (AV). In the authors' experience these first-line systemic antibiotics for acne, help reduce pruritus in AV. Studies on human keratinocytes have shown that doxycycline may have greater effect in this aspect, compared to erythromycin.

Patients with mild-to-moderate acne based on the Comprehensive Acne Severity Scale (CASS) and associated itch intensity of more than 2 on a 10-point numerical scale were recruited. The 29 subjects were eligible to be part of the study, out of them 14 received erythromycin while 15 received doxycycline. At baseline and at 6 weeks after treatment, an itch questionnaire assessing the average itch intensity over the prior 1 week on a 10-point numerical scale, frequency of itch (graded 1–7, ranging from 1 episode a month to more than 10 episodes daily) and itch quality-of-life assessment (16 questions, each graded 1–6 ranging from not affected to severely affected, giving a total score of 16–96) was given to the subjects. The severity of acne was also graded by a dermatologist blinded to the treatment arm based on CASS, at baseline and at 6 weeks. Analyses were performed on a per-protocol basis using the paired t-test and two-sample t-test.

Statistically significant reduction in itch intensity scores at 6 weeks was seen with doxycycline, and not with erythromycin. But the difference between the two, in reducing itch intensity scores, was not statistically significant. The itch QOL scores were significantly better in both groups but the frequency of itch was not much different.

There were no previous reports of the anti-pruritic efficacies of systemic antibiotics in the treatment of acne. The efficacy of doxycycline in this regard maybe due to reduction in inflammation and attenuation of the protease-activated receptor 2 interleukin-8 pathway. A limitation of this study is the relatively high dropout rate (19%) and small sample size. It is concluded from this study that doxycycline effectively reduces itch intensity in pruritic acne and this effect was independent of improvements in acne severity. Doxycycline may serve as a good antibiotic option for patients who experience itch in their acne lesions.

Key Messages
- Doxycycline attenuates the protease-activated receptor 2 interleukin-8 axis in the modulation of proinflammatory responses hence reduces itch
- Effectively reduces itch intensity in pruritic acne and may serve as a good antibiotic option for patients who experience itch.

ARTICLE 58

Does Isotretinoin Cause Depression and Anxiety in Acne Patients?

Metekoglu S, Oral E, Ucar C. Does isotretinoin cause depression and anxiety in acne patients? *Dermatol Ther.* 2019;32(2):e12795.

Abstract

The aim of this article is to research the effect of isotretinoin treatment on depression in a group of patients undergoing isotretinoin therapy. Behavioral tests measuring anxiety and depression, and the measures assessing acne severity and quality of life (QOL) were applied to 112 acne patients. A significant decrease was observed in Hospital Anxiety Depression Scale-depression (HAD-D), Hospital Anxiety Depression Scale-anxiety (HAD-A), Global Acne Grading System (GAGS), and Cardiff Acne Disability Index (CADI) scores at the end of the therapy. There was no significant relationship between patients depression history and HAD-D scores at the end of the first month of therapy and at the end of treatment. Although the psychiatrists are concerned about the potential psychiatric side effects of isotretinoin, there is no causal relationship between isotretinoin use and depression in acne patients.

COMMENT

This article is a prospective study to assess the effect of isotretinoin treatment on depression in patients undergoing treatment with isotretinoin for acne. Acne has been associated with adverse psychiatric symptoms. In dermatology outpatient clinics, approximately 25.2% of patients with acne experience some psychiatric morbidity. Few studies have evaluated the clinically significant diagnostic category of major depressive disorder among people with acne.

There are several treatment options for acne based on its severity. Isotretinoin, a synthetic oral retinoid has great efficacy against moderate-to-severe acne. Isotretinoin is only indicated for acne when it is severe and does not respond to oral or topical antibiotic or topical retinoid (recalcitrant acne) or for acute-onset severe acne with systemic complaints (acne fulminans). Since its introduction, many adverse psychiatric effects, including depression, violent behavior, psychosis, suicide, mood swings, and suicide attempts were reported. Most of the dermatology-based studies point to the lack of evidence-relating depression to isotretinoin use. However, a causal relationship has not yet been established, and the link between isotretinoin use and psychiatric events remains controversial.

In this article, 112 acne patients who had nodulocystic acne or treatment resistant forms of acne (papulopustular, cystic, and conglobated) were studied. Routine laboratory tests, including complete blood count and differential, serum blood lipid measurements, liver enzyme tests (and a pregnancy test for women of child-bearing age) were obtained before treatment. The patients were asked specific questions about history of depression and family history of depression.

Acne severity by Global Acne Grading System (GAGS), quality of life (QOL) by Cardiff Acne Disability Index (CADI), anxiety, and depression by Hospital Anxiety Depression Scale (HAD) at baseline, at the end of the first month of therapy and at the end of treatment were assessed. The results of this study indicate that there was no increase in HAD-D and HAD-A scores in acne patients who were treated with isotretinoin. At the end of therapy, there was a significant decrease in HAD-D scores. This study reveals that successful treatment of acne with isotretinoin improves HAD-D, HAD-A, GAGS, and CADI scores at the end of therapy.

Though more than three decades have passed since the first report in 1983 linking isotretinoin with depression; this issue is still debatable. Overall, case reports, database studies, and retrospective studies show a possible association between isotretinoin and depression. Prospective studies, however, on the other hand, show no association or, in some studies, improvement of depressive symptoms.

Although few psychiatrists are concerned about depressive effects of isotretinoin use, their data support no causal relation between isotretinoin use and depression. Most of acne patients who had HAD-D scores above 7 and/or HAD-A scores above 10 in the course of treatment consulted to the psychiatrist were not diagnosed as depression. Hence, isotretinoin treatment should not be refused automatically to patients with a history of depression.

Key Messages

- Isotretinoin is the most powerful drug amongst the various drugs used for its treatment. A causal relationship has not yet been established between isotretinoin use and depression
- Successful treatment of acne with isotretinoin improves quality of life and HAD-D scores, hence isotretinoin treatment should not be refused automatically to patients with a history of depression.

ARTICLE 59

Treatment of Atrophic Acne Scarring with Fractional Micro-plasma Radiofrequency in Chinese Patients: A Prospective Study

Lan T, Xiao Y, Tang L, et al. Treatment of atrophic acne scarring with fractional micro-plasma radio-frequency in Chinese patients: a prospective study.
Laser Sur Med. 2018;50(8):844-50.

Abstract

Fractional micro-plasma radiofrequency is a novel technology that produces minor ablation to the epidermis to promote rapid reepithelialization, while the radiofrequency evoked thermal effect can stimulate regeneration and remodeling of dermal fibroblasts. A total of 95 patients with facial atrophic acne scars were treated by micro-plasma radiofrequency using three sessions at 2-month intervals. There was a significant improvement in acne scars after three treatments. This can be an effective and safe treatment for acne scars, and might be a good choice for patients with darker skin.

COMMENT

Acne scarring is a common complication of moderate-to-severe acne. Atrophic acne scarring on face can have a severe negative effect on psychological well-being and quality of life (QOL) of patients. Though various techniques are available for atrophic acne scars, they have different risks of adverse side effects. Fractional micro-plasma radiofrequency technology is a recent modality that makes use of a discharge of radiofrequency energy acting on a stream of nitrogen gas very close to the surface of the skin by spicules on the roller. The radiofrequency energy triggers micro-sparks in the plasma between the skin surface and the spicules of the handpiece which cause mild epidermal ablation and perforate the dermis superficially to form microchannels. These micro-channels can be used to increase penetration of the drug such as recombinant human basic fibroblast growth factor (Rh-bFGF), to promote the wound healing and collagenesis. Being suitable for Asians with darker skin types, it has a variety of indications.

Ninety-five Chinese patients with moderate-to-severe degree of atrophic facial acne scarring, with Fitzpatrick skin types III or IV were enrolled in this study. All patients received three treatment sessions at 2-month intervals using the micro-plasma radiofrequency device (Pixel RF, Accent XL; Alma Lasers, Caesarea, Israel) and were reviewed 6 months after the last treatment. In every session, the lesions were treated with three to four passes in different directions of the roller tip under topical EMLA (eutectic mixture of local anesthetics). The rh-bFGF was applied to the treated area to promote the lesion re-epithelialization. Patients were asked to score their pain level on a point scale from 0 to 10 (0 1/4 no pain and 10 1/4 extremely painful) based on visual analogue scales (VAS) after each treatment. All patients were instructed to avoid contact with water and scratching for 3–5 days after each treatment. Patients also were asked to use SPF 50 sunscreen with a sun protection after epithelialization had taken occurred.

Échelle d'Evaluation Clinique des Cicatrices d'Acné (ECCA) scores were used to quantify acne scar improvement. Three dermatologists who were not part of the treatment evaluated the improvement of facial atrophic acne scars based on photographs taken before the first treatment and 1, 3, and 6 months after the last treatment and they were blinded about the photos being pre- or post-treatment. Clinical response was graded using the following scale—none (no improvement, 0), mild (<25% improvement, 1), moderate (25–50% improvement, 2), good (51–75% improvement, 3), and excellent (>75% improvement, 4). The possible side effects seen were scaling, infection, pain, erythema, edema, effusion; scar formation, and dyschromia were recorded.

The acne scars of all patients showed objective improvements at the last follow-up (100% response rate); the improvement in the lesion was graded as excellent in 17.44% (15/86), good in 53.49% (46/86), moderate in 27.90% (24/86), and mild in 1.16% (1/86). The mean ECCA score reduced to 47.27 from 107.21 ($p < 0.05$), 6 months after the last treatment all patients showed improvement in large pores, spots, UV spots, texture, red areas, porphyrin fluorescence ($p < 0.05$) compared with baseline. At 6-month follow-up, an obvious improvement was observed. No patients were dissatisfied at the clinical response of the treatment for atrophic acne scars. The 2.44 was the average score for satisfaction for improvement of acne scars at last follow-up. There were no serious adverse effects during the treatment and follow-up visits. Pain after treatment was a common complaint. Other side effects were edema, erythema, scaling, and effusion.

The results revealed the fractional microplasma radiofrequency is an effective and safe method for the treatment of atrophic acne scars. It can also improve spots, red areas, active acne lesions, large pores, texture, UV spots, and possibly even wrinkles within the treatment area. Clinical studies in the future should explore different methods of alleviating this pain by using a forced cool air chiller before treatment, or performing plasma treatment under general anesthesia.

Key Messages

- Fractional microplasma radiofrequency has been introduced as a dual function modality in dermatology
- It can produce a microablative effect promoting rapid skin re-epithelialization, along with a thermal effect stimulating regeneration and remodeling of dermal fibroblasts. It is an effective and safe method for the treatment of atrophic acne scars.

ARTICLE 60

Comparison of Novel Dual Mode versus Conventional Single Pass of a 1450-nm Diode Laser in the Treatment of Acne Vulgaris for Korean Patients: A 20-week Prospective, Randomized, Split-face Study

Kwon HH, Choi SC, Jung JY, et al. Comparison of novel dual mode versus conventional single pass of a 1450-nm diode laser in the treatment of acne vulgaris for Korean patients: a 20-week prospective, randomized, split-face study. *J Cosmet Dermatol. 2018;17(6):1063-8.*

Abstract

The 1450-nm diode laser incorporating dynamic cooling device (DCD) has been shown to be effective for treating acne and hyperseborrhea, along with dermal remodeling effects. This wavelength sufficiently penetrates deeply to thermally affect the infra infundibulum and sebaceous glands. This conventional 1450-nm diode laser high-energy stamp-only regimen is often associated with pain and hyperpigmentation, especially in dark-skinned individuals. This study aimed to evaluate the novel dual regimen with conventional regimen for acne treatment in Asian patients. The dual mode side demonstrated better improvements in both inflammatory and noninflammatory lesion counts, acne severity assessments, and reduction in sebum secretion compared with Stamp only conventional regimen.

COMMENT

The 1450-nm diode laser incorporating dynamic cooling device (DCD) has been shown to be effective for treating acne and hyperseborrhea. The presumed mechanism in vivo is through heating of the sebaceous gland and associated structures, subsequently leading to the impairment of sebaceous gland activity and associated inflammation. The standardized treatment regimen has not been fully established in particular for Asian patients. A conventional stamping regimen, applying each shot around the whole face with energies from 12 J/cm^2 to 16 J/cm^2, has frequently caused severe pain and discomfort, even with the concurrent use of DCD, in addition, to postinflammatory hyperpigmentation, especially in dark-skinned individuals.

The present study was aimed to evaluate a novel regimen sequential application of low energy (5-7 J/cm^2) stamp mode to inflammatory lesions only, followed by 4-5 passes of moving mode over the full face. A 20-week, prospective, randomized split-face protocol to compare clinical aspects for acne treatments between two facial sides receiving the 1450-nm diode laser novel dual mode versus conventional single pass. Twenty-five Korean subjects Fitzpatrick skin type III to V with acne underwent three sessions 4 weeks apart and assessed subjectively and objectively at 12 weeks post the last session. Inflammatory, noninflammatory acne and seborrhea were significantly reduced more in the dual mode group. Pain scores were significantly lower in the dual mode group as also the erythema and edema. No postinflammatory hyperpigmentation was observed in the dual mode side. Thus, the dual mode appears to be safer and more effective than the conventional single pass mode. Relatively longer exposure with lengthened pulse duration may effectively decrease sebaceous gland activity compared with target only based approaches. In addition, lower fluence with DCD off in this method definitely decreases the incidence of side effects. The limitations being, all patients were of the same ethnic background, histopathologic analysis for various markers for lipogenesis and inflammation was not done and long-term maintenance beyond 3 months was not evaluated.

Key Messages

- The diode laser, (especially in the dual mode,) is a viable option for acne treatment either as monotherapy or as combination therapy, overcoming major limitations of the other more ubiquitous treatments for acne patients
- In the dual mode, one low fluence energy shot is administered selectively for each inflammatory acne lesion with the stamp mode. Then gentle linear movement of laser hand piece as in laser toning along full facial area is followed for 4–5 passes after switching to the moving mode. This relatively longer exposure with lengthened pulse duration may effectively decrease sebaceous gland activity compared with the conventional mode with decreased side effects especially in dark skinned individuals.

ARTICLE 61

Resurfacing of Facial Acne Scars with a New Variable-pulsed Er:YAG Laser in Fitzpatrick Skin Types IV and V

Chathra N, Mysore V. Resurfacing of facial acne scars with a new variable-pulsed Er:YAG laser in Fitzpatrick skin types IV and V.
J Cutan Aesthet Surg. 2018;11(1):20.

Abstract

The aim of the study was to check efficacy and safety of the new variable square pulse (VSP) Er:YAG laser in the management of acne scar in patients with Fitzpatrick skin types IV and V. The newer modified Er:YAG, equipped with variable pulse duration technology, promises to bridge the gap between a conventional Er:YAG laser and CO_2 laser. This retrospective study consisted of 80 patients who had undergone four treatment sessions with VSP technology equipped with Er:YAG laser, using a combination of ablative and fractional mode, to improve acne scars with minimal risks and downtime.

COMMENT

This is a retrospective study on the effectiveness and safety of VSP Er:YAG laser in acne scar management in Fitzpatrick skin type IV and V. The Er:YAG laser, (considered to be less effective than CO_2 laser in its traditional form), has a new modulated form with VSP technology, alters the pulse width and energy simultaneously, offering a superior way to control the degree of ablation and deep tissue heating maximizing patient safety by minimizing excess laser energy absorption into the surrounding skin. The microshort pulse (MSP) mode of nonfractionated Er:YAG was used in ablating hypertrophic scars and raised borders of scars. Fractional Er:YAG, in Short Pulsed and Long Pulsed mode, was used for the depressed center of the scars to stimulate neocollagenesis. The Turbo mode, allows multiple rapid applications of a beam to a single spot, thus increasing the ablation depth of the original beam.

Eighty patients had undergone four sittings of Er:YAG laser treatment. The outcome was assessed both subjectively and objectively at the end of four sessions. Subjective scoring was based on the photographic assessment by the observer and patient satisfaction and objective scoring was done using Goodman and Baron's Qualitative and Quantitative global scarring grading systems. Significant number of patients slipped down a grade or two as per qualitative grading system. All 80 patients had a drop in the total quantitative score at the end of four sessions with significant drop in mean score. However, the perceived subjective improvement by patients was more than that of observers. A quarter of patients also had reduction in pores. It was most effective in treatment of rolling and superficial box car type of scars. However, patients with predominantly ice pick scars did not show significant improvement. Prolonged erythema, crusting and post inflammatory hyperpigmentation lasting 1 month were observed in 1 or 2 patients only.

Due to the superior tissue dynamics and side effect profile, the variable-pulsed Er:YAG using a combination of ablative and fractional mode can effectively may prove to be more useful than the earlier versions of this laser, both in safety and efficacy.

Key Messages
- Variable-pulsed Er:YAG laser is an advantage as it allows the largest range of thermal depth control and therefore the most complete range of treatments
- Er:YAG in longer pulse duration, mimics CO_2 laser in inducing collagen contraction and coagulation of small dermal vessels and is most useful for base of atrophic scars
- Short pulse duration produces superficial ablation with minimal thermal effect, like conventional Er:YAG laser. Therefore, the short pulse mode can be used to smooth the scar borders and in hypertrophic scars
- It can be potentially as effective as fractional CO_2 laser with better safety profile in Fitzpatrick skin types IV and V.

ARTICLE 62

A Novel Topical Minocycline Foam for the Treatment of Moderate-to-severe Acne Vulgaris: Results of 2 Randomized, Double-blind, Phase 3 Studies

Gold LS, Dhawan S, Weiss J, et al. A novel topical minocycline foam for the treatment of moderate-to-severe acne vulgaris: results of 2 randomized, double-blind, phase 3 studies.
J Am Acad Dermatol. 2019;80(1):168-77.

Abstract
Acne vulgaris (AV) is a chronic inflammatory disease with inflammatory and noninflammatory lesions. The first-line therapy for patients with moderate-to-severe acne is oral minocycline. Topical formulation of minocycline confers the advantages of enhanced bioavailability with less systemic toxicity. This article is a clinical trial in phase 3 program, consisting of 2 identical double-blind trials and a 40-week open-label phase, initiated to investigate the efficacy and safety of topical minocycline FMX101 4% in the treatment of moderate-to-severe AV.

COMMENT

Acne vulgaris (AV) is a chronic inflammatory skin disease characterized by inflammatory lesions (papules, pustules, and nodules) and noninflammatory lesions (blackheads and whiteheads). Acne is associated with significant impairment of quality of life (QOL) leading to anxiety and depression. Treatment depends on the grade of acne. Oral antibiotics are indicated in moderate-to-severe acne but have limited usage due to its resistance. Tetracyclines are less susceptible to resistance, with minocycline having the lowest resistance rate with its antibacterial and anti-inflammatory activity. Systemic acne therapy may have lower adherence rates than topical therapy, potentially because of dissatisfaction arising from the lack of efficacy and the occurrence of side effects. A topical formulation of minocycline was expected to confer the advantages of facilitated local application and enhanced bioavailability while providing the drug's proven high efficacy in acne.

A pharmacokinetic study of topical once-daily minocycline FMX101 4% for up to 21 days demonstrated no significant systemic absorption. Hence with statistically significant and clinically meaningful improvement in phase 2 trial with a favorable safety in moderate-to-severe acne patients, clinical phase 3 trial of Topical minocycline FMX101 4%, a double-blinded randomized study was conducted to investigate the efficacy and safety of topical minocycline.

Its (double-blind, multicenter; 30 sites), vehicle-controlled studies, Study 04 (NCT02815267) and study 05 (NCT02815280) were identical and randomized for age 9 years or older in moderate-to-severe facial acne. Use of oral retinoids or corticosteroids within 12 weeks and topical retinoids, topical anti-inflammatory drugs and corticosteroids, oral antibiotics, or other systemic acne treatment within 4 weeks before randomization was prohibited.

These eligible subjects applied topical minocycline FMX101 4% foam once daily for 12 weeks in the evening. Efficacy and safety were assessed at weeks 3, 6, 9, and 12. At week 12, subjects continued into the open-label phase for an additional 40 weeks. Absolute change in inflammatory lesion counts from baseline and the rates of IGA on the IGA scale (Investigator's Global Assessment) assessed treatment success.

Only 1% of the subjects had adverse events, FMX101 4% showed superior efficacy to vehicle in reducing both inflammatory and noninflammatory lesions (co-primary end point) from baseline in both studies. Reductions in inflammatory lesions were evident as early as week 3 with FMX101 4% in both studies and maintained until the end of treatment. It potentially lower risk of systemic side effects and improves the treatment adherence. Though the foam delivery system for topical drugs is easy to apply and does not leave a greasy or oily film, this study has limitations. This include duration of 12-week study may not be adequate to demonstrate the long-term safety profile of topical minocycline and lack of an active comparator arm.

> **Key Messages**
> - Topical tetracyclines, with their potent antibacterial and anti-inflammatory activity and potentially minimal systemic side effects, are an unmet need for acne therapy
> - Once-daily, FMX101 topical minocycline foam 4% appears to be safe, well tolerated, and effective in treating moderate-to-severe acne; minocycline foam represents an important treatment option for patients with acne.

ARTICLE 63

Management of Comedonal Acne Vulgaris with Fixed-combination Topical Therapy

Gold MH, Baldwin H, Lin T. Management of comedonal acne vulgaris with fixed-combination topical therapy. J Cosmet Dermatol. 2018;17:227-31.

Abstract

Acne vulgaris (AV) is a common chronic inflammatory disease of the skin. Clinically, it is characterized by a combination of open and closed comedones, papules and pustules. While comedonal acne is typically the mildest form of the disease, it can be the hardest to treat as comedones are usually firmly seated within the follicle. Topical retinoids have long been advocated for the treatment of comedonal acne. The present study reviews the benefits seen with fixed combinations with and without retinoids.

COMMENT

Treatment guidelines have traditionally advocated the use of topical retinoids to treat comedonal acne. All topical retinoids effectively reduce the number of comedones as well as inflammatory lesions in mild-to-moderate facial acne. Acne is a chronic inflammatory disease and early inflammatory events lead to development of the microcomedo, hence several studies are evaluating the response of comedonal acne to combination treatment with topical retinoids and topical dapsone having additional antibacterial and anti-inflammatory properties. These combination therapies appear to enhance the efficacy against comedonal acne relative to the use of the retinoid alone. Benzoyl peroxide (BPO) is an important component in combination therapy, as it reduces the development and emergence of antibiotic-resistant to *Propionibacterium acnes*.

English language literature review was performed using Medline, EMBASE, and the Web of Science, and relevant articles were reviewed to know the latest data on the use of fixed-combination topical therapy in comedonal acne. The combinations compared in this article are topical retinoids with BPO, topical clindamycin with BPO, topical clindamycin with retinoids and the additive effect of dapsone and clindamycin/BPO to retinoid therapy. The combination of topical retinoid with agents that also have direct or indirect anti-inflammatory properties has been found to be more effective in reducing comedonal acne given importance of inflammation in the pathogenesis of acne. This suggests that combination therapy is the best choice. Few comparative studies show that adapalene 0.1%-BPO 2.5% gel has comparable results to clindamycin 1%-BPO 5% gel, and adapalene 0.3%-BPO 2.5% gel. Meta-analysis suggests that clindamycin 1.2%-BPO 2.5% gel was more effective than clindamycin benzoyl peroxide 5% gel in noninflammatory lesions, and similar studies suggest additional benefits of higher doses of BPO (3.75% vs. 2.5%) in this fixed combination.

Key Messages
- Topical retinoids alone have been recommended for the treatment of comedonal acne lesions
- Fixed-combination therapy has been shown to be more effective than individual agents as they have direct or indirect anti-inflammatory properties.

ARTICLE 64

Blunt Cannula Subcision is more Effective than Nokor Needle Subcision for Acne Scars Treatment

Gheisari M, Iranmanesh B, Saghi B. Blunt cannula subcision is more effective than Nokor needle subcision for acne scars treatment.
J Cosmet Dermatol. 2019;18(1):192-6.

Abstract
The objective of this study was to compare the effectiveness of Nokor needle subcision (NNS) and blunt cannula subcision (BCS), for treatment of acne scars. Blunt cannula subcision had better outcomes with lesser or milder complications and single session treatment when compared with conventional (NNS) surgery.

COMMENT

Acne scars not only affect the appearance of a person but also affect the mental and social well-being. Many methods have been introduced in the past that attempts to enhance the therapeutic effect and reduce the complications. Most common treatments for acne scars include the following—punch excision, punch elevation, subcision, laser skin resurfacing, elliptical excision, skin graft, and tissue augmentation. The side effects and inflammatory responses make the Nokor needle subcision (NNS) outcome and efficacy questionable. Blunt cannula has been proposed as a potentially proper alternative for Nokor needles, and others have implied that cannula may be more efficient in treating acne scars based on its efficacy for treatment of cellulite.

In the present split-face study, subcision using Nokor needle and blunt cannula have been compared in 34 patients with rolling type of atrophic scars. Patients were blinded about the therapeutic method of treatment on each malar area. The procedure was done under tumescent anesthesia (1 mL epinephrine in 1,000 mL normal saline + 10 mL bicarbonate + 50 mL lidocaine) with one side using Nokor needle and blunt cannula at the another side. Post subcision antibiotic prophylaxis was given. Complications included ecchymosis and nodule formation after NNS or only edema after BCS procedures.

Patients and physician satisfaction rates were compared at one and three months. Patients were significantly satisfied with blunt cannula subcision (BCS) but not with NNS, during 3-month monitoring. Physician-1 was satisfied with both BCS and NNS outcome however, the satisfaction rate was higher for BCS, after 3 months than 1-month monitoring. Physician-2 was only significantly satisfied with NNS at 3 months than 1-month visits however, satisfaction percentages were higher in BCS treated than NNS-treated sides. It implies that cannula subcision is a safe method with high efficacy and patient's satisfaction because of single perforation instead of multiple injections in other methods which reduces the patient's pain and risk of scars. Furthermore, treatment sessions and recovery time will be reduced compared to most of other conventional methods. Thus BCS can be a promising treatment modality for atrophic rolling type of acne scars.

Key Messages
- *Subcision procedure using blunt cannula could be an acceptable substitute for Nokor needle when treating rolling scars*
- *Blunt cannula subcision has promising outcomes including lesser or milder complications and single session treatment instead repeating perforations compared with other conventional surgery-based methods for acne scar remediation.*

ARTICLE 65

Novel Tretinoin 0.05% Lotion for the Once-daily Treatment of Moderate-to-severe Acne Vulgaris in a Preadolescent Population

Eichenfield LF, Sugarman JL, Guenin E, et al. Novel tretinoin 0.05% lotion for the once-daily treatment of moderate-to-severe acne vulgaris in a preadolescent population.
Pediatr Dermatol. 2019;36(2):193-9.

Abstract

The aim of this study was to evaluate the safety and efficacy of once-daily tretinoin 0.05% lotion in preadolescent subjects (≤13 years) with moderate-to-severe acne. The analysis of two multicentric, trials in moderate-to-severe acne was considered. Inflammatory and noninflammatory lesions in preadolescent acne reduced significantly with tretinoin 0.05% as compared to vehicle. It was well-tolerated, with no major adverse events.

COMMENT

One of the first signs of pubertal maturation is preadolescent acne (≤13 years). Topical retinoids are commonly used to treat acne; safety and efficacy are well documented in large published trials. With limited FDA approved treatment options for preadolescent acne, off-label prescribing is common. Monotherapy with tretinoin microsphere gel, tretinoin gel, and adapalene gel, has been investigated in small open label and blinded studies in children under 12 years of age. However, data in preadolescent acne are lacking. In a posthoc analysis of two studies comparing tretinoin microsphere 0.1% gel and tretinoin 0.05% gel in adolescents (10-14 years) with mild-to-moderate acne, comparable lesion reduction and treatment success were noted. Tretinoin 0.05% gel is better tolerated.

A new lotion formulation of tretinoin 0.05% has recently been developed leveraging polymerized emulsion technology with the aim to improve both efficacy and tolerability of tretinoin. This was a posthoc analysis of two identical multicenter, randomized, double-blind, vehicle-controlled, parallel group clinical studies in pediatric subjects with moderate-to-severe acne. Preadolescent subjects (n = 154) randomized (1:1) to receive tretinoin 0.05% lotion or vehicle, once daily for 12 weeks. Efficacy assessments included changes in baseline and subsequent study visits (weeks 4, 8, and 12) of inflammatory/noninflammatory lesions and treatment success [at least 2-grade reduction in Evaluator's Global Severity Score (EGSS) and clear/almost clear]. Additional assessments included a Patient Satisfaction Score (PSS) and a validated Acne-specific Quality of Life (Acne-QOL) Questionnaire. Safety, adverse events (AEs) and cutaneous tolerability was evaluated throughout.

Tretinoin 0.05% lotion has shown to provide significantly greater efficacy than vehicle in two phase 3 studies. At week 12, mean percent reduction in noninflammatory and inflammatory lesion counts were 49.5% and 44.0% compared with 31.4% and 18.8% with vehicle (both p = 0.001). Treatment was successful in 23.7% of subjects by week 12, compared with 7.2% (p = 0.009) in vehicle. The majority of AEs were mild and transient—most frequently were application site pain (5.6%) and application site dryness (2.8%). Local cutaneous safety and tolerability assessments were generally mild-to-moderate and improved by week 12. Results in this pediatric population were comparable to those seen in the overall study populations. The only difference was that the vehicle tended to be less effective in the pediatric population. In the overall study populations, tretinoin 0.05% lotion showed significantly greater QOL benefits relative to vehicle.

Tretinoin 0.05% lotion is a novel topical treatment for moderate-to-severe acne leveraging polymerized emulsion technology. It was developed to provide a tretinoin formulation with improved tolerability and efficacy that could be especially suited to a preadolescent population. The polymerized emulsion forms a mesh (a polymeric network) which helps structure the emulsion providing uniform distribution of hydrating and active ingredients at the surface of the skin, thus reducing the presence of concentrated drug in specific areas (hot spots). It forms a barrier which helps keep the skin moist by reducing epidermal water loss and increasing skin water content. Tretinoin 0.05% lotion offered significantly more efficacy than vehicle in reducing the lesions, with higher patient satisfaction (compared with vehicle) and preference (compared with previous acne therapy). Efficacy in comedonal acne was similar to that reported previously with tretinoin microsphere 0.04% gel.

Tretinoin 0.05% lotion formulation is an effective and well-tolerated topical treatment for moderate-to-severe comedonal and inflammatory preadolescent acne.

Key Messages

- Tretinoin 0.05% lotion is a novel topical treatment for moderate-to-severe acne leveraging polymerized emulsion technology
- The polymerized emulsion provides a mesh which helps structure the emulsion providing uniform distribution of active and hydrating ingredients at the surface of the skin, reducing the presence of concentrated drug in specific areas.

ARTICLE 66

Efficacy of Two Plant Extracts Against Acne Vulgaris: Initial Results of Microbiological Tests and Cell Culture Studies

Kılıç S, Okullu SÖ, Kurt Ö, et al. Efficacy of two plant extracts against acne vulgaris: Initial results of microbiological tests and cell culture studies.
J Cosmet Dermatol. 2018.

Abstract

The effect of plant extracts on gene expression levels of IL-1α, SRD5A1, and TNFα in HaCaT cells was observed. Anti-acne extract 1 (AE1) consisted of *Juglans regia* (walnut husk), *Myrtus communis* (myrtle leaves), *Matricaria chamomilla* (chamomilla flowers), *Urtica dioica* (stinging nettle leaves), and *Rosa damascena* (rose flowers). Anti-acne extract 2 (AE2) contained *Brassica oleracea var. botrytis* (broccoli) and *Brassica oleracea var. italica* (cauliflower). The action on two different strains of *Propionibacterium acnes* was studied. Human keratinocyte cells were used for in vitro tests. The RT-qPCR was used for gene analysis. Strong antibacterial and anti-inflammatory activities were demonstrated by both the extracts. In conclusion, the topical application of these botanical extracts can be good candidates for local acne treatment.

COMMENT

Acne vulgaris (AV) is a common skin disease that results from the androgen-induced increased sebum production, inflammation, altered keratinization, and colonization of *P. acnes* on the pilosebaceous follicles. The main consideration in the development of acne is the androgen-induced overproduction of sebum along with hypertrophy of sebaceous glands. As antibiotics are the common therapeutic agents, emerging antibiotic resistance in bacteria is certainly a threat for effective treatment. Thus, there is a prominent need for alternative treatment methods. There are studies in the literature that indicate the anti-inflammatory and antibacterial effects of certain botanical extracts against acne in humans. This study evaluates the antimicrobial efficiency of the extracts against *P. acnes* and the effects of the extracts on the gene expression levels of IL-1α, SRD5A1, and TNFα in HaCaT cells.

Anti-acne extract 1 containing *M. communis, J. regia, M. chamomilla, U. dioica,* and *R. damascena* showed both anti-inflammatory activity and high antimicrobial activity against *P. acnes*. While phenolic substances of *J. regia* such as chlorogenic acid, caffeic acid, ferulic acid, catechin, vanillic acid, and juglone show antioxidant activity, particularly herbaceous juglone (5-hydroxy 1,4-naphthoquinone) exhibits antimicrobial properties. The water extract of *M. communis* leaves showed a significant antibacterial effect against *Escherichia coli, Staphylococcus epidermidis, Salmonella typhimurium,* and *Pseudomonas aeruginosa. Matricaria chamomilla* is composed of therapeutically active compounds such as sesquiterpenes, flavonoids (apigenin, rutin) coumarins, and polyacetylenes, bisabolol. Bisabolol isolated from essential oils could reduce inflammation, fever, adjuvant arthritis, yeast-induced fever in rats. Apigenin exhibited anti-inflammatory activity in carrageenan-induced rat paw edema and delayed-type hypersensitivity in mice. The ethanolic extract of *M. chamomilla* has also antibacterial and antifungal effects. *Urtica dioica* were a source of kaempferol, myricetin, linoleic acid, oleic acid, iron, and beta-sitosterol. Polysaccharides and caffeic malic in all parts of *U. dioica* showed anti-inflammatory activity. *Rosa damascena* contains flavonoids such as kaempferol and quercetin and their glycoside derivatives, carboxylic acids terpene, myrcene, tannins, and vitamin C. The hydroalcoholic extract of *R. damascena* was effective in reducing inflammatory pain.

Anti-acne extract 2 was composed of *B. oleracea L var. italica* and *B. oleracea var. botrytis*. The presence of glycosides, alkaloids, carbohydrates, tannins, flavonoids and proteins in *B. oleracea* is associated with antibacterial and anti-inflammatory activities.

In the gene expression analysis, AE1 increased the expression level of TNFα (1.1719, $p < 0.0001$), suppressed the expression level of IL-1α, SRD5A1 (0.0588, $p = 0.0231$; 0.3081, $p = 0.0351$), respectively. AE2 suppressed gene expression level of IL-1α, SRD5A1, TNFα (0.3815, $p = 0.0254$; 0.3418, $p = 0.0271$; 0.1997, $p = 0.0623$).

Both plant extracts demonstrated strong anti-inflammatory effects and antibacterial activity against *P. acnes*. Further studies are needed to characterize the active components within these extracts associated with these properties and thus conduct more focused studies in the path of new drug development.

Key Messages

- Antibiotic is in the center of antimicrobial treatment, emerging antibiotic resistance in bacteria is certainly a threat for effective treatment. Thus, there occurs a prominent need for alternative treatment methods
- Both plant extracts demonstrated strong anti-inflammatory effects and antibacterial activity against *P. acnes*.

ARTICLE 67

Female Type of Adult Acne: Physiological and Psychological Considerations and Management

Dréno B, Bagatin E, Blume Peytavi U, et al. Female type of adult acne: Physiological and psychological considerations and management.
J Dtsch Dermatol Ges. 2018;16(10):1185-94.

Abstract

Adult female acne has a distinct clinical presentation with a number of specific pathophysiological features and gender-specific triggers. Psychological distress is much greater in adults compared to adolescents. Also, the impact of disease is greater for female patients, triggering higher levels of psychosocial anguish and increasing the likelihood of sequelae such as skin picking and the risks of cutaneous superinfection, scarring and postinflammatory hyperpigmentation (PIH), and acne recurrence. A comprehensive, holistic approach to the patient as a whole encompassing the medical symptoms, individual lifestyle factors and the impact of acne on her quality of life (QOL) is required.

COMMENT

Acne vulgaris (AV) usually regresses during the late adolescence or early adulthood. There are three subtypes of acne among those who experience acne after adolescence—(1) persistent acne (a continuation of the disease from adolescence into adulthood); (2) relapsing acne, with regression after adolescence and recurrence in adulthood; and (3) late-onset acne, which first presents well after puberty (commonly in the early- to mid-twenties). The specific characteristics of adult female acne include:

- Acne on chin deep-seated, long lasting small nodules (<0.5 cm) and cysts in the U zone
- Mixed presentations with both inflammatory and noninflammatory lesions are also common
- Truncal acne is less common
- Hyperseborrhea is present in 70% of patients
- Flare-ups before menstruation are seen in about half of adult patients with acne and appear to be more common in older women.

There are three main pathophysiological factors—(1) resistant strains of *Propionibacterium acnes* may initiate and exacerbate inflammatory lesions; (2) levels of dehydroepiandrosterone sulfate (DHEA-S) in the upper range of normal stimulate IL-2 production and enhance Th1 immune function, and (3) a genetic predisposition in over half the patients. There is also elevated levels of anti-Müllerian hormone and increased serum levels of insulin-like growth factor 1. They can be hence treated by low-glycemic-load dietary restrictions.

Adult acne is easy to diagnose, but some conditions have similar presentations and should be excluded, including grade 2 rosacea (flushing and inflammatory lesions), *Staphylococcus aureus* folliculitis, boils, syringomas, milia, acne agminata, *Demodex* folliculitis, *Pityrosporum* folliculitis, and perioral dermatitis.

Adult acne has a greater psychological impact due to a prolonged course. Factors that influence the psychological impact of acne include judgments of others, perceived sexual attractiveness, stress, relationships with family and friends, stigmatization, and fear of scarring or disease persistence. A holistic approach is required while managing women with acne, considering the features like severity extent, and duration of disease; response to previous treatments; predisposition to scarring and postinflammatory hyperpigmentation (PIH), including patient preference, mindset and lifestyle (comprising personal relationships, sun tanning, nutrition, family planning, smoking, professional life and sporting activities) and sensitivity of the skin.

Retinoids are the first-line choice for most mild-to-moderate types of adult acne. Azelaic acid (20% cream or 15% gel) is also used as the first-line choice for mild-to-moderate adult acne, can be used even in pregnant women. Benzoyl peroxide (BPO) has strong bactericidal properties and is safe in pregnancy. With mild inflammatory acne, topical retinoids can be combined with azelaic acid, BPO, sytenol or clindamycin phosphate in fixed formulations.

Systemic treatments are usually required for moderate-to-severe acne as well as for mild forms (mainly mandibular acne) associated with scarring, long duration or failure to respond to topical therapies. Systemic antibiotics like doxycycline, minocycline and lymecycline are preferred choices but tetracyclines and retinoids need to be avoided during pregnancy. Hormonal therapies, including third/fourth generation oral contraceptives (OC) and anti-androgens primarily reduce excess sebum production and should be used in combination. Metformin can be used off-label to decrease insulin resistance. Spironolactone as low-dose monotherapy (50-150 mg/day) or combined with topical therapy can be used for resistant cases. (A third/fourth generation OC may be added for menstrual irregularity); adrenal androgen inhibitors (low-dose glucocorticoids, e.g. prednisone) are recommended for acute flares and short-term treatment of severe acne or androgenic disorders. Isotretinoin is specifically indicated for use after failure of other therapies; however, in women, it may be used as first-line treatment for severe nodular cystic acne or second-line treatment for severe acne unresponsive to topical/oral combination therapy. Maintenance therapy is required to minimize the risk of relapse after acute treatment and where recurrences are frequent. Psychological evaluation is generally only undertaken in secondary care or if the psychological effect of acne is regarded as particularly severe.

Key Messages

- *Adult acne has specific clinical and pathophysiology*
- *Psychological impact of acne can be greater in women than female adolescents due to a more persistent course, despite a presentation that is usually less severe*
- *The management of adult female acne should encompass not just medical treatment of the symptoms, but also a comprehensive, holistic approach to the patient as a whole, her individual lifestyle factors and the impact of acne on her quality of life.*

ARTICLE 68

The Efficacy and Safety of Nonpharmacological Therapies for the Treatment of Acne Vulgaris: A Systematic Review and Best-evidence Synthesis

De Vries FM, Meulendijks AM, Driessen RJ, et al. The efficacy and safety of nonpharmacological therapies for the treatment of acne vulgaris: a systematic review and best-evidence synthesis.
J Eur Acad Dermatol Venereol. 2018;32(7):1195-203.

Abstract

Pharmacological therapy is not always desirable because of the development of antibiotic resistance or the potential risk of adverse effects. Nonpharmacological therapies can be viable alternatives for conventional therapies. This is a systematic review to assess the efficacy and safety of several nonpharmacological therapies in the treatment of acne vulgaris. Circumstantial evidence was found for nonpharmacological therapies in the treatment of acne vulgaris. However, the lack of high methodological quality among included studies prevented the authors from drawing clear conclusions.

COMMENT

This systematic review assesses the safety and efficacy of nonpharmacological therapies like chemical peels, laser and light-based therapies, dermabrasion microneedling, (micro) and (mechanical) lesion removal in the treatment of acne vulgaris. Three electronic databases (MEDLINE, Cochrane library, CINAHL) were used to search for studies on nonpharmacological therapies for acne vulgaris, published between January 2000 and May 2017. Inclusion criteria were as follows: nonpharmacological therapies, studies on participants with acne vulgaris, split-face designs and parallel group designs, randomized controlled trials (RCTs) and controlled clinical trials (CCTs), control group designs, all stages and phases of acne severity, all acne outcome tools, studies that were exclusively performed in humans and studies that were published in English, Dutch or German. Exclusion criteria were as follows: pharmacological therapies (except when served as a control intervention), studies reported on acneiform dermatoses other than acne vulgaris, acne scars, studies combining several therapies (e.g. photodynamic therapy), surgical procedures, experimental therapies, studies without a control group, studies that were unavailable in full text and studies with home use devices,. Two reviewers independently screened all studies and selected potentially relevant studies that met the inclusion and exclusion criteria. Both reviewers resolved any differences of opinion on whether or not to include a particular study by consulting a third reviewer (Driessen).

The primary outcome was changed in the clinical signs of inflammatory lesions and noninflammatory lesions, reported through relative values (percentage improvement of acne compared to baseline), absolute values (the number of acne lesions or sebum level), or by an ordinal level (based on acne grading scales). The secondary outcome of interest was safety of nonpharmacological therapies, reported as tolerability and (adverse) side effects. Total 1,467 studies were identified, out of which 33 eligible studies (1,404 participants) met the inclusion criteria and were included in the systematic review. Safety of three main nonpharmacological therapies in the treatment of AV—chemical peels, laser- and light-based therapies, and fractional microneedling radiofrequency (FMRF) were evaluated. Although a high rate of statistically significant results was found in most of the studies, indicating efficacy of nonpharmacological therapies, the low methodological quality of the included studies made it difficult to draw clear conclusions. Strong evidence of the treatment efficacy for glycolic acid (10-40%) was demonstrated, whereas moderate evidence was found for amino fruit acid (20-60%), IPL (400-700 and 870-1,200 nm) and the diode laser (1,450 nm). The most frequently reported side effects for nonpharmacological therapies included tolerable pain, erythema, edema and a few cases of hyperpigmentation, which were in most cases mild and transient. The strict application of inclusion and exclusion criteria led to the exclusion of several studies on other frequently applied nonpharmacological therapies, such as (micro)dermabrasion and mechanical lesion removal (mostly due to the absence of a control group).

An important limitation of this review is the high level of heterogeneity among included studies. These variabilities could have possibly given rise to the contradictory findings concerning the photodynamic light therapy. Another limitation of this study is the scarce data on the treatment with FMRF. First, the small sample size gave rise to non-statistically significant results. The short follow-up periods showed that these results may not be applicable for the effects on long-term treatments. There was high risk of bias among the majority of the studies. The most common risk of bias noted was performance bias. The research integrity was unclear in most studies, such as possible conflict of interest, a commercial sponsorship by the intervention supplier (especially for laser devices, FMRF devices or chemical peels), which might have introduced some bias in the results too. This systematic review found circumstantial evidence for nonpharmacological therapies in the treatment of AV. This review indicates a great interest in this topic, which lay emphasis on the need for further research, using double-blind placebo-controlled study designs with a homogeneous data collection and processing.

Key Messages

- A strong evidence of the treatment efficacy was seen with glycolic acid (10–40%), moderate evidence was found IPL and the diode laser and conflicting evidence was found for PDL therapy
- Most frequently reported side effects for nonpharmacological therapies included erythema, tolerable pain, edema and a few cases of hyperpigmentation, which were in most cases mild and transient.

ARTICLE 69

Clindamycin Phosphate 1.2%/Benzoyl Peroxide 3% Fixed-dose Combination Gel versus Topical Combination Therapy of Adapalene 0.1% Gel and Clindamycin Phosphate 1.2% Gel in the Treatment of Acne Vulgaris in Japanese Patients: A Multicenter, Randomized, Investigator-blind, Parallel-group Study

Kawashima M, Hashimoto H, Alió Sáenz AB, et al. Clindamycin phosphate 1.2%/benzoyl peroxide 3% fixed-dose combination gel versus topical combination therapy of adapalene 0.1% gel and clindamycin phosphate 1.2% gel in the treatment of acne vulgaris in Japanese patients: A multicenter, randomized, investigator-blind, parallel-group study. *British J Dermatol. 2015;172(2):494-503.*

Abstract

Combinations of adapalene 0.1% (ADA) with clindamycin phosphate 1.2% (CLNP) (ADA + CLNP) and the fixed combination of CLNP and benzoyl peroxide 3% (CLNP/BPO 3%) are commonly recommended for the early treatment of acne vulgaris (AV) in Japan. This article compares clinical efficacy and safety of the above two regimens in the treatment of AV. CLNP/BPO 3% showed greater efficacy for the early treatment of AV in Japan, with a more favorable safety profile than ADA + CLNP.

COMMENT

Acne vulgaris (AV) is a common skin condition affecting males and females of various ages worldwide, with a global prevalence of 9.4%. Proliferation of *Propionibacterium acnes* in the microcomedo leads to local inflammation. Acne therapies can be classified as—intervention treatments that target the characteristic inflammatory and noninflammatory lesions (IL and non-IL); maintenance treatments which help prevent disease relapse and adjunctive therapies which aim at disease sequelae, such as scars and postinflammatory hyperpigmentation. The aim of this study was to compare the early efficacy and safety of CLNP (clindamycin phosphate)/BPO (benzoyl peroxide) 3% with Japanese standard topical use of ADA (adapalene) + CLNP in the treatment of AV.

This was a phase IV, multicenter study. About 351 patients of facial AV were randomized to receive CLNP/BPO 3% or ADA + CLNP for 12 weeks. Patients with nodulocystic acne, those on topical corticosteroids or other systemic therapy for acne were excluded. Patients were assessed at screening (baseline) and at weeks 1, 2, 4, 8, and 12 of treatment. CLNP/BPO 3% or ADA gel was applied once a day before bedtime, covering the entire face. CLNP was only applied to lesion in the morning and after applying ADA in the evening. The primary result was to evaluate change from baseline in the total lesion (TL) counts at week 2. Secondary end-points included the percentage change from baseline in TL, Investigator's Static Global Assessment (ISGA), inflammatory and noninflammatory lesion (IL and non-IL) counts, quality of life [QOL (Skindex-16)] and patient preference. Local tolerability scores and adverse events were also recorded.

Once-daily application of the CLNP/BPO 3% gel was found to be more efficacious than the topical combination of ADA + CLNP at reducing TL at week 2 and also IL from week 2 onward (but not non-IL). There has been a synergistic antibacterial activity of BPO and tertiary amines such as CLNP. Treatment with CLNP/BPO 3% improved patient QOL to a greater extent than did ADA + CLNP as per Skindex-16 assessments. Inability to blind participants and shorter time duration limits this study. There was no significant difference in TL at week 8 and 12 between the treatment groups. This may reflect the different onset of action with respect to IL between BPO (earlier efficacy onset of action) and ADA (slower efficacy onset of action). A higher incidence of facial adverse drug reactions (ADR) in the ADA + CLNP group was noted. CLNP/BPO 3% was well-tolerated, and patients reported better QOL and patient-preference scores compared with those using ADA + CLNP. These results support the strong recommendation of CLNP/BPO 3% as a first-line treatment of patients with AV in the current Japanese guidelines.

Key Messages

- The CLNP/BPO 3% would be more effective compared with ADA + CLNP, especially in the treatment of IL during the early stage
- The CLNP/BPO 3% combination gel contains two active ingredients that have antibacterial effects, which is responsible for early reduction in acne lesions and improvement in acne severity
- This study strongly recommends of CLNP/BPO 3% as a first-line treatment of patients with acne vulgaris in the current Japanese guidelines.

ARTICLE 70

Screening of Body Dysmorphic Disorder in Acne Patients: A Pilot Study

Marron SE, Gracia-Cazana T, Miranda-Sivelo A, et al. Screening of body dysmorphic disorder in acne patients: a pilot study. 2019;110(1):28-32.

Abstract

Body dysmorphic disorder (BDD) is a condition in which the patient feels ugliness about his looks which is disproportionate to the physical defect. Its onset is seen in early adolescence. As acne is also a disease of adolescence, BDD can coexist in this subject. Hence this article analyzed the prevalence of BDD in acne patients. It was observed that BDD was prevalent in 8.6% patients of mild acne and 14.8% in moderate acne patients. Hence these patients should be screened with simple BDD questionnaire to detect early and refer for further management.

COMMENT

Body dysmorphic disorder (BDD) is a mental health condition in which the patient will have subjective feeling of ugliness and patient believes that any minor physical defect which is within normal parameters is very evident to others. Although BDD onset is in adolescence, it is diagnosed later in life because patients are ashamed to talk about their symptoms. The prevalence of BDD in general population is 2, in adolescents it is 3.6% however in dermatological practice it is up to 10–12%. Acne is one such dermatological condition which has several links with BDD. Both have their onset in adolescence. Skin especially facial skin a frequently involved site for acne mainly determines the body image. BDD, tanning behaviors and compulsive acne excoriation often coexist. This prospective and observational study analyses the prevalence of BDD in acne patients. All patients fulfilling inclusion and exclusion criteria were subjected to BDD questionnaire derived from Diagnostic and Statistical Manual of Mental Disorders, Fourth Edition (DSM-IV) criteria for BDD. Two criteria were used to identify BDD cases one was positive result in Body Dysmorphic Disorder Questionnaire with four positive points and a negative exclusion question and the other was cook acne grading score that included most stringent criteria with mild/non-noticeable lesions and least stringent criteria with moderate lesions. The analysis revealed that BDD was prevalent in 8.6% when the most stringent criteria were used and 14.8% when least stringent criteria were applied. Patients with BDD spent approximately 2 hours a day thinking about their appearance. BDD should be kept in mind while treating patients with acne for early detection and referred to psychiatric care.

Key Messages
- The BDD and acne both having onset in adolescence may coexist together
- Patients with acne should be screened for early detection of BDD for further management.

ARTICLE 71

A Qualitative Investigation of the Impact of Acne on Health-related Quality of Life: Development of a Conceptual Model

Fabbrocini G, Cacciapuoti S, Monfrecola G. A qualitative investigation of the impact of acne on health-related quality of life (HRQL): development of a conceptual model.
Dermatol Ther. 2018;8(1):85-99.

Abstract

The article analyzes qualitative investigation of the impact of acne on health-related quality of life (HRQOL) and aims at development of a conceptual model. It demonstrates that moderate-to-severe acne has an extensive impact on adolescents' and adults' HRQOL. The study also aimed to determine the attributes of topical treatments for acne that are the most important for patients. Accordingly, participants preferred a gel formulation, room temperature storage, application with fingers, and a once-daily regimen.

COMMENT

Although acne is not life-threatening or physically disabling but can have significant negative impact on the quality of life (QOL) of the affected individuals. As compared to quantitative research, qualitative research allows an in-depth investigation into patients' experiences. It helps to identify concepts important to patients, in terms of HRQOL impact and experience of using treatment for acne. This qualitative data is used to develop conceptual models to illustrate the impact of a condition and hypothesize links between the concepts.

The study involved adolescent and adult acne patients on topical medication who were subjected to semi-structured interview guides based on the literature review of HRQOL in acne. The interviews included series of sociodemographic, clinical questions and open-ended questions to allow participants to spontaneously describe the ways in which acne affects them and about different areas of HRQOL.

The analysis showed that emotional functioning, social functioning, relationships, leisure activities, daily activities, sleep, and school/work were significantly affected in acne patients. There was reduced self-confidence or self-esteem thus hindering participation in school activities and socializing. Feeling isolated or lonely was reported in adults with acne. It also affected social interaction and the use of social media. Feeling of discomfort, embarrassed, anxious, or intimidated was reported when talking to new people. It also affected leisure activities like swimming and sports/exercise. Acne medication consumed their day to day time and type of clothing was also modified by the site of acne. One-third of the adolescents also reported disturbed sleep. It also hindered overall performance at school and work in few. With all these the authors developed a conceptual model of the impact of acne on HRQOL. Conceptual models can be useful tools that provide a visual representation of the impact of a condition, allowing the links between concepts to be identified.

Participants in the study preferred a gel formulation, room temperature storage, application with fingers, and a once-daily regimen for better compliance.

Key Messages
- Acne significantly affects emotional functioning, social functioning, relationships, leisure activities, daily activities, sleep, and school/work
- Patients prefer a gel formulation, room temperature storage, application with fingers, and a once-daily regimen for better compliance.

ARTICLE 72

Host-microbiome Interactions and Recent Progress into Understanding the Biology of Acne Vulgaris

O'Neill AM, Gallo RL. Host-microbiome interactions and recent progress into understanding the biology of acne vulgaris. *Microbiome. 2018;6(1):177.*

Abstract
The article throws insight into the newer pathophysiological mechanisms in the development of acne. It reviews recent developments in the interactions of skin microbes with host immunity, discussing the contribution of dysbiosis to the immunobiology of acne and newly emerging skin microbiome-based therapeutics to treat acne.

COMMENT

The article discusses mainly the synergistic and competitive interactions between cutaneous microbes and its effect on host immune responses relevant to acne vulgaris (AV). An exciting area of recent advances within the understanding of acne has resulted from studies focused on the skin "microbiome," the complex community of bacteria, viruses, and fungal organisms that inhabit all epithelial surfaces and appear to have distinctive functions on the skin. Though *C. acnes* has been implicated as a causative organism, no convincing evidence exists to suggest bacterial overgrowth corresponds to acne development or disease severity. Recent research with tools to visualize *C. acnes* colonization in the in vivo setting has shown biofilms attached to the hair shaft extending from the stratum corneum to the base of the follicle. They have reported more *C. acnes* biofilms in acne lesions compared to control follicles. Populations of *Staphylococcus*, *Cutibacterium*, and *Malassezia* form the composition of these biofilms. The interactions between these species dictate biofilm phenotype, and also contribute to enhanced antibiotic resistance and inflammatory capacity. A biofilm matrix acts as a biological glue to physically restrict sebum passage into the infundibulum, leading to comedo formation and/or promote retention and accumulation of corneocytes in the lumen, resulting in a keratinaceous plug and comedone development. A recent study compared the skin microbiome of acne patients using three different sampling techniques—pore strips, swab, and gel biopsy combined with multiple sequencing approaches the authors concluded that surface or follicular sampling were both suitable approaches for accurate analysis of the skin microbiome in acne research, particularly in the context of *C. acnes* association.

Typing methods involving cell wall sugar analysis, serological agglutination, bacteriophage, and fermentation profiling have revealed three distinct *C. acnes* phenotypes called type I, II, and III. *C. acnes* type I class can be subdivided into closely related subtypes: IA1, IA2, IB, and IC, that contain many different clonal complexes (CC) and Sequence Types (ST)s. It is shown that one ST18 among the phylotype IA1 was globally disseminated and related with severe acne that several ST's from CC72 (type II) and CC77 (type III) were associated with healthy skin.

Metagenomics analysis of *C. acnes* has shown that the 3 most abundant ribotypes (RT1, RT2, RT3) are evenly distributed among both acne and normal follicles, four ribotypes including RT4 and RT5 of the phylotype IA1 were significantly higher in 30-40% of patients with acne, but rarely found in individuals with healthy skin, however, RT6 which represents a subpopulation of phylotype II was found to be 99% associated with healthy skin.

In another metagenomic analysis of acne patients, higher relative abundance of *C. granulosum* in healthy individuals was observed as compared to acne thus stressing upon the role of commensals. However, further investigations are required to determine the contribution of this minor *Cutibacterium* species.

A dynamic shift by colonization by *C. acnes* in the microenvironment of the follicle triggers inflammation by production of proinflammatory cytokines IL-12 and IL-8 due to host antimicrobial peptides (AMP) play a role in the pathogenesis of acne.

Researchers have also found genomic alterations in *C. acnes* species from healthy and acne skin. Although it remains unclear if these single genetic elements drives pathogenesis of a multifactorial disease like acne. According to gene ontology analysis, the most significant biological process in acne skin was "response to bacterium." The most common bacterial proteins found being *C. acnes*. The interaction between various bacteria alters the host response. In acne, the microbial dysbiosis could be due to androgen-mediated seborrhea and dysseborrhea.

This article also discusses several new microbiome-targeted strategies that are in trial. One such modality is application of a suspension of *Nitrosomonas eutropha*, an ammonia-oxidizing bacteria (AOB), isolated from organic soil samples. It exploits the bacterium's nitrogen cycle to convert ammonia and urea, to nitrite and NO, which have anti-inflammatory and antimicrobial activity. NO has known to have a dual role, one directly killing *C. acnes* and also suppressing cytokine release in keratinocytes.

The research on probiotics and prebiotics suggests that the gut–brain–skin axis, posits a mechanism that connects gastrointestinal health by oral probiotics to skin homeostasis. It is shown that pre and probiotics reduce systemic markers of oxidative stress, inflammation, regulate inflammatory cytokine release in the skin, improving skin barrier function and hydration.

Heat-killed *C. acnes* (HKCa)-based vaccine and vaccine targeting the cell wall-anchored sialidase or the secreted CAMP factor 2 are under trial.

Key Messages
- It is now well-established that *C. acnes* phylotype IA1 is associated with acne, while types II and III isolates are more commonly associated with healthy skin
- Microbial dysbiosis is known to have a significant role in acne pathogenesis
- New research aims at addressing these microbiota.

ARTICLE 73

Acne in Lomé, Togo: Clinical Aspects and Quality of Life of Patients

Saka B, Akakpo AS, Téclessou JN, et al. Acne in Lomé, Togo: clinical aspects and quality of life of patients. *BMC Dermatol.* 2018;18(1):7.

Abstract

The article assesses the quality of life (QOL) in patients with acne. It also aims to determine if there is any correlation between the QOL and the severity of acne. The questionnaire-based study showed that acne significantly affects the QOL and there is a positive correlation between the severity of acne and DLQI scores.

COMMENT

Acne has a significant psychological impact affecting the quality of life (QOL) in these patients. In this article, the acne patients included in the study were subjected to clinical examination and were graded with ECLA (Échelle de Cotation des lésions d'acné) scale. CADI (Cardiff Acne Disability Index) scale were calculated based on the questionnaire which included five items to evaluate the emotions of the patient, his social relations, the avoidance behaviors, feelings of anxiety, and the overall perception of acne. ECLA and CADI scored were then correlated to know the relation between the severity of acne and its impact on the QOL.

The analysis showed that QOL was impaired in all patients and also there was a positive and significant correlation between the severity of acne and impairment of patients' QOL. Even minimal acne can have a negative impact on QOL. They found a positive correlation between the CADI score and factors like type, intensity of facial acne and the presence of scars. These factors significantly influence QOL impairment. It was also observed that acne in areas apart from the face did not have much impact on the QOL as the lesions were hidden. It was also observed a positive correlation between the severity of acne and patient relations, avoidance behaviors, overall perception of acne and anxiety triggered by acne.

Key Messages
- Acne had a negative impact on the QOL of patients which is directly proportional to severity of acne
- Acne has an impact on the patient's relationships, avoidance behaviors and overall perception of acne.

ARTICLE 74

The Role of the Physician in Patient Perceptions of Barriers to Primary Adherence with Acne Medications

Ryskina KL, Goldberg E, Lott B, et al. The role of the physician in patient perceptions of barriers to primary adherence with acne medications.
JAMA Dermatol. 2018;154(4):456-9.

Abstract

Nonadherence to acne treatment is a major hindrance in the management of acne. In this study, the factors involved with nonadherence were evaluated. A qualitative analysis was conducted from structured interviews with patients reporting nonadherence with acne medications. Physician-level interventions to improve primary adherence to medications for acne may have an impact on nonadherence with costly medications, although they may not affect patient satisfaction with the prescribing physician.

COMMENT

Though nonadherence is common, little is published about modifiable factors associated with primary nonadherence to acne medications. The objectives of this study were to—(1) understand patient perceptions of barriers to primary adherence to acne medications, (2) describe patient perceptions of physicians' role in alleviating or exacerbating those barriers, and (3) identify modifiable factors to improve primary adherence.

Structured interviews were conducted with patients who were prescribed acne medications by a dermatologist but however did not initiate treatment. This included patients who did not submit the prescription to pharmacies, did not collect the medication, or picked up the medication but did not use it. Nonadherence was assessed through patient self-report during recruitment.

Recent trends in insurance coverage and medication prices may have led to higher out-of-pocket costs, especially in dermatology. The authors observed that though patients were concerned about out of- pocket costs of prescribed acne medications, they did not discuss costs with physicians. Interventions to improve primary adherence should incorporate discussion of medication costs and provide specific alternative plans in case the patient is unable to fill the prescription, rather than asking patients to call back.

Future studies should evaluate the prevalence of these barriers to primary medication adherence for acne. Medication prices were the main reason that most patients did not initiate recommended acne treatments. Despite anticipating insufficient insurance coverage, patients were reluctant to deal with the considerations with physicians and generally did not expect physicians to be knowledgeable in this area. Whereas this experience did not appear to negatively affect satisfaction with the physicians, physicians who discuss medication costs and provide a concrete alternative plan may be able to improve primary adherence among their patients.

Key Messages
- Patients are concerned about out-of- pocket costs of prescribed acne medications
- Physicians who discuss medication costs and provide a concrete alternative plan may be able to improve primary adherence among their patients.

ARTICLE 75

Exploring the Relationship between Stress and Acne: A Medical Student's Perspective

Maleki A, Khalid N. Exploring the relationship between stress and acne: a medical student's perspective. *Clin Cosmet Investig Dermatol. 2018;11:173.*

Abstract

The aim of this cross-sectional questionnaire-based study was to assess the role of stress in the severity of acne in medical students who themselves are subjected to high level of stress. This article also tries to establish the effectiveness of stress-reduction techniques in students via selected components in controlling acne. It also aids in distinguishing whether the stress leading to acne originates from extrinsic factors or individual's "intrinsic" predisposition to produce the stress response.

COMMENT

Acne is known to negatively affect the quality of life (QOL) and mood, so it is possible that acne can lead to stress and stress, in turn, aggravating acne. The author recommends that stress and acne levels in students should be measured at different times during the medical course and values relative to each individual to be compared. The author emphasizes the effects of stress-reducing techniques on acne severity. The role of lifestyle factors, such as exercise and sleep, on stress and acne should be evaluated in future studies just not only in females but males too.

Key Messages

- *Acne is a common disorder with significant psychological impact*
- *Stress is known to aggravate acne lesions and stress-reducing techniques have an adjuvant and important role in acne management.*

ARTICLE 76

The Impact of Acne and Facial Postinflammatory Hyperpigmentation on Quality of Life and Self-esteem of Newly Admitted Nigerian Undergraduates

Akinboro AO, Ezejiofor OI, Olanrewaju FO, et al. The impact of acne and facial post-inflammatory hyperpigmentation on quality of life and self-esteem of newly admitted Nigerian undergraduates.
Clin Cosmet Investig Dermatol. 2018;11:245.

Abstract

Acne and facial postinflammatory hyperpigmentation are relatively common clinical conditions among adolescents and young adults, and inflict psychosocial injuries on sufferers. This study was conducted on newly admitted undergraduates. Acne with facial hyperpigmentation induces poorer quality of life (QOL) and self-esteem is impaired only in severe acne. Beyond the medical treatment of acne, dermatologists should routinely assess the QOL and give attention to treatment of facial postinflammatory hyperpigmentation among people of color.

COMMENT

Acne leads to psychosocial complications, which in turn, have implications on quality of life (QOL), vocational and academic performance, and self-esteem. The presence of postinflammatory hyperpigmentation (PIH) induced by acne is a cause of additional distress among acne patients. PIH amplifies already impaired psychosocial status, and is associated with the use of cosmetic camouflage due to imperfections. Acne and its accompanying blemishes have been related to embarrassment, depressive symptoms, feeling of uselessness, poor self-attitude, reduced pride, self-worth and body dissatisfaction in adolescent late teenage years.

This was a cross-sectional study done on newly admitted undergraduates in Nigeria. The study participants completed questionnaire to obtain their history, including their present age, ageat acne onset, pus discharging acne eruptions history of facial itch, painful acne eruptions, and the presence of acne related PIH. The participants were asked regarding their feelings about the presence of acne and its complications, including whether or not they felt stigmatized, socially unacceptable, ashamed, judged, depressed, anxious or emotionally upset by their acne. In the present study, in addition, to mild-to-moderate acne, about 56.0% of the participants presenting with acne had some degree of facial PIH. The presence of acne related PIH was significantly associated with a feeling of frustration, aggression and embarrassment among young acne sufferers. They also described social avoidance and negative feelings about their appearance.

Special attention should be given to the treatment of PIH in acne patients, as without this the QOL would not improve, because PIH contributes significantly to its impairment. Although there was no distinction in the self-esteem of participants with acne and hyperpigmentation and those without it, male self-esteem was significantly affected. The present study is restricted as it is hospital-based and might not be representative of the general population from which sampling was drawn. Beyond the treatment of acne, PIH should be treated in people of color to improve their QOL. Appropriate referral to a psychologist is necessitated when QOL and self-esteem are impaired.

Key Messages
- Acne and PIH have been related to depressive symptoms, embarrassment, feeling of uselessness, poor self-attitude, reduced pride, self-worth and body dissatisfaction in adolescents
- Beyond the treatment of acne, PIH should be treated in people of color to improve their QOL.

ARTICLE 77

Which Acne Treatment has the Best Influence on Health-related Quality of Life? Literature Review by the European Academy of Dermatology and Venereology Task Force on Quality of Life and Patient Oriented Outcomes

Chernyshov PV, Tomas Aragones L, Manolache L, et al. Which acne treatment has the best influence on health-related quality of life? Literature review by the European Academy of Dermatology and Venereology Task Force on Quality of Life and Patient Oriented Outcomes.
J Eur Acad Dermatol Venereol. 2018;32(9):1410-9.

Abstract
European Academy of Dermatology and Venereology (EADV) Task Forces (TF) performed a literature search on Quality of Life and Patient Oriented Outcomes (QOL and PO) in Acne, Rosacea and Hidradenitis Suppurativa (ARHS), and found most of the publications were health-related (HR) QOL. Members of the EADV TF on QOL and PO decided to detect which acne treatment has the best influence on HRQOL of acne patients. So a new literature search was performed to find publications on acne treatment where the HRQOL of patients was assessed as an outcome measure. Dermatology-specific and acne-specific instruments showed much better sensitivity to successful therapeutic intervention than generic HRQOL instruments. The most frequently used HRQOL instrument was the dermatology life quality index (DLQI) questionnaire.

COMMENT

Guidelines are meant to describe a systematic treatment escalation based on disease severity and treatment response; starting with topical treatments using, e.g. benzoyl peroxide (BPO) or retinoids, progressing over systemic therapies with antibiotics to isotretinoin. Adopting a quality of life (QOL) measure as an integral part of acne management was recommended by the European Dermatology Forum S3-Guideline for the Treatment of Acne. Generic, dermatology and disease-specific QOL instruments were used as outcome measures to assess the efficacy of different treatment methods. The highest numbers of studies identified were those concerning isotretinoin and BPO. Members of the EADV TF on QOL and PO decided to detect which acne treatment has the best influence on HRQOL of acne patients. Authors of the position paper on QOL measurement in acne were invited to participate. All those who volunteered were allocated a section of the identified articles to review.

The new word "quimp", meaning the QOL impairment, was recommended for routine clinical and research use. More than half of the studies were funded by pharmaceutical companies, 16 papers had no information about funding, authors of two studies reported no industrial support and one study was supported by the noncommercial organization. Norethindrone acetate/ethinyl estradiol-treated subjects experienced greater (statistically significant) improvements in all four domains of the Acne-QOL when compared with placebo-treated subjects. Studies which compare different treatments with the same duration and HRQOL instrument are important to establish treatment options with the best effect on patients' HRQOL. The improvement in total dermatology life quality index (DLQI) score for the 5% BPO two times a day group was significantly less than for all the other groups. The acne-symptoms domain of the Acne-QOL showed a greater improvement ($p = 0.002$) for patients using adapalene 0.1% and BPO 2.5% fixed-dose combination gel and oral doxycycline compared to patients using the gel vehicle and oral doxycycline. Responses to individual DLQI questions were significantly lower in the adapalene group than the tretinoin group.

The use of the mean change of HRQOL impairment after the treatment makes it possible to identify which acne treatment method had the best effect on HRQOL. Comparing the impact of different treatment methods on HRQOL of patients assessed by the same instrument is a more methodologically reliable approach but in the case of high diversity of instruments and a lack of well-designed studies, it also leads to significant limitations. According to the results of double-blind, randomized comparative studies, the highest changes of HRQOL from baseline were reported with regard to patients treated with isotretinoin (measured by the DLQI) 15 and BPO/clindamycin topical gel (measured by the Acne-Q4).

Oral isotretinoin showed the highest HRQOL change (measured by the DLQI) in open-label multiple group studies. Oral isotretinoin, topical clindamycin phosphate 1% gel/BPO 2.5%, oral norethindrone acetate/ethinyl estradiol, and adapalene 0.1%/BPO 2.5% fixed-dose combination gel showed better effect on HRQOL than placebo. Oral isotretinoin caused the most prominent improvement of acne impact in the studies where HRQOL was measured. Acne-specific instruments may assess HRQOL in both children and young adults, dermatology-specific instruments have established age limits. There is a limited number of high-quality studies on acne treatment where HRQOL were assessed. No high-quality studies on acne treatment with less than 8 weeks duration were found. The EADV TF on QOL and PO recommends to present numeric data on HRQOL before and after treatment in all studies where HRQOL instrument are used as outcome measures.

> **Key Messages**
> - Generic, dermatology and disease-specific QOL instruments were used as outcome measures to assess the efficacy of different treatment methods
> - The EADV TF on QOL and PO recommends to present numeric data on HRQOL before and after treatment in all studies where HRQOL instrument are used as outcome measures.

ARTICLE 78

Stressful Life Events and Psychiatric Comorbidity in Acne–A Case Control Study

Bondade S, Hosthota A, Basavaraju V. Stressful life events and psychiatric comorbidity in acne–a case control study. *Asia Pac Psychiatry. 2019;11(1):e12340.*

Abstract

This study was performed on one hundred patients with acne vulgaris in the age group of 12–45 years. Age- and sex-matched controls were taken. Sociodemographic details were collected using a semi-structured proforma. The Presumptive Stressful Life Event Scale (PSLES) was used to assess stressful life events. Anxiety was evaluated using the Hamilton Anxiety Rating Scale (HAM-A) and depression by the Hamilton Depression Rating Scale (HAM-D). The undesirable stressful life events and psychiatric comorbidity were found to be more in acne patients than in controls.

COMMENT

This research was conducted to evaluate the relationship of stressful life events, psychiatric comorbidity and acne. This was a hospital-based cross-sectional case-control study undertaken at medical college in Bangalore for a duration of 3 months. One hundred successive patients who were diagnosed with acne vulgaris (AV) in the age group of

12–45 years were included. Subjects were given a semi-structured proforma to collect sociodemographic details. Acne was graded taking into account the predominant lesions and stressful events were collected using the presumptive stressful life event scale (PSLES). Psychiatric diagnosis was made according to the Diagnostic and Statistical Manual 5 (DSM-5) criteria; depression, by using Hamilton Depression Rating Scale (HAM-D) and anxiety was assessed using the Hamilton Anxiety Rating scale (HAM-A).

In this study, stressful life events were observed in 89 patients and 92 controls, which was not statistically important. In 65 patients with acne and 50 controls, the undesirable life occurrences were present, this distinction was statistically important. However, there was no significant difference between the groups with respect to desirable and ambiguous life events. This observation suggests that life events do not affect the severity of the acne but may play a part in flaring of acne. The most prevalent stressful life event in patients with acne was getting married or appearing for examinations. In this study, change of eating habits was the second most common stressful life event, followed by excessive use of alcohol by a family member, and transfer or change of working conditions; conflict with in-laws or broken affair were more in patients than in controls.

During periods of emotional stress, there is an increased release of corticotrophin-releasing hormone, glucocorticoids, and adrenal androgens that up-regulate sebocyte conversion of androgen precursors to testosterone induced sebaceous hyperplasia and can have a negative impact on cutaneous permeability. Stress would lead to inhibition of epidermal lipid synthesis, wound healing, and compromise in antimicrobial defense that could delay the repair of acne lesions. When life events were compared in subjects having psychiatric comorbidity, the undesirable life events were more in patients having acne than in controls.

Psychosomatic strategy for patients with psychiatric comorbidity is suggested for patients with acne, which involves stress management, relaxation sessions, instructional programs and suitable medication. Psychotherapy helps an individual to reinterpret events and develop strategies to cope with a stressful event. There are certain limitations in this study. It was a hospital-based cross sectional study with small sample size and hence cannot be generalized.

Key Messages

- *Getting married or appearing for exams were the most common stressful life event in acne patients*
- *Psychosomatic approach, which includes stress management, relaxation sessions, educational programs and appropriate medication for patients having psychiatric comorbidity, is recommended for patients having acne.*

ARTICLE 79

The Evaluation of Psychiatric Comorbidity, Self-injurious Behavior, Suicide Probability, and other Associated Psychiatric Factors (Loneliness, Self-esteem, Life Satisfaction) in Adolescents with Acne: A Clinical Pilot Study

ÖzyayEroğlu F, Aktepe E, Erturan İ. The evaluation of psychiatric comorbidity, self-injurious behavior, suicide probability, and other associated psychiatric factors (loneliness, self-esteem, life satisfaction) in adolescents with acne: a clinical pilot study.
J Cosmet Dermatol. 2019;18(3):916-21.

Abstract

In this study, psychiatric comorbidity and levels of self-injurious behavior, suicide probability, life satisfaction, self-esteem and loneliness in adolescents with acne was assessed and compared with a control group. The presence of high levels of psychiatric comorbidity, suicide probability, and self-injurious behavior in adolescents with acne in this study suggests that psychiatric evaluation should be included in acne treatment plans. Multidisciplinary approach for acne treatment is important.

COMMENT

Psychologically, adolescents are more volatile and prone to change in appearance. For this reason, acne can lead to the development of emotional and behavioral reactions such as deterioration in body perception, decline in self-esteem, shame, loneliness, anger, inward closure and psychiatric disorders beyond cosmetic anxiety. Although acne vulgaris (AV) is known to have negative effects on both mental and emotional state of the person, there is no study in the literature that examines the relationship between AV and self-injurious behavior (SIB).

In this research, one to one clinical psychiatric assessment in adolescents with AV explored psychiatric comorbidity, the likelihood of suicide, SIB, and other associated psychiatric variables, and the information were compared with a control group. Acne quality of life scale (AQLS), Life Satisfaction Scale (LSS), University of California Los Angeles (UCLA) Loneliness Scale, Rosenberg Self-Esteem Scale, Suicide Probability Scale (SPS), Turkish version of the Schedule for Affective Disorders and Schizophrenia for School-Age Children-Present and Lifetime version (aged 6-18 years) (K-SADS-PL-T), and SIB evaluation inventory were applied to all participants.

A psychiatric comorbidity has been discovered in the present research in 37.5% of adolescents with acne. Psychiatric comorbidity was found to be significantly higher in adolescents with acne than in adolescents without acne, and psychiatric diagnoses were found to increase when the quality of life (QOL) of the individuals with acne was lower. In addition, among the adolescents with a psychiatric comorbidity, those with acne had significantly lower self-esteem, lower life satisfaction and higher loneliness levels than adolescents without acne. The most commonly identified diagnoses were post-traumatic stress disorder (PTSD), generalized anxiety disorder (GAD), major depressive disorder (MDD), and bulimia nervosa (BN). The most common type of SIB in the adolescents with AV was preventing wound healing, followed by hair break, tucking and pinching behaviors.

The most significant restriction is that the pattern of the research was cross-sectional and by self-report some of the results were acquired. In conclusion, AV should not be treated only as a cosmetic problem but also as a mental health problem and routine psychiatric evaluations should be included in the treatment plan.

Key Messages
- Acne can lead to the development of emotional and behavioral reactions such as deterioration in body perception, decrease in self-esteem, shame, loneliness, anger, inward closure and psychiatric disorders beyond cosmetic anxiety
- The most commonly identified psychiatric diagnoses were generalized anxiety disorder, post-traumatic stress disorder, major depressive disorder, and bulimia nervosa.

ARTICLE 80

Acne Relapses: Impact on Quality of Life and Productivity

Dreno B, Bordet C, Seite S, et al. Acne relapses: impact on quality of life and productivity. (Registre Acné'Dermatologists). Acne J Eur Acad Dermatol Venereol. 2019;33(5):937-43.

Abstract
This non-interventional, real-life study investigated the rate of acne relapses, and their impact on the quality of life and productivity (loss/absenteeism) among teenagers and adults. The Global Acne Severity (GEA) Scale was applied for homogenous assessment of acne severity. Cardiff Acne Disability Index (CADI), SF12-physical score (PS) and SF12-mental score (MS) questionnaires were used for quality of life assessments. Acne relapses were significantly associated with impaired quality of life and productivity loss/absenteeism.

COMMENT

There are two kinds of acne in female adults, "persistent acne", which is a disease continuation from adolescence, representing approximately 80% of instances of adult acne and "late-onset acne" which first occurs at adulthood, representing approximately 20%. Acne exposome is the sum of all environmental factors influencing acne occurrence, duration and severity. These exposome factors may be classified into six categories—nutrition, medication, occupational factors, pollutants, climatic factors and psychological and lifestyle factors. Upon multivariate analysis, acne relapse was a significant determinant of absenteeism/productivity loss. Independently of acne severity and other variables, those suffering from relapses were found more likely to miss work/school.

Further study on acne relapses should concentrate on better characterizing the group of patients experiencing more psychological distress or absenteeism and may require further help from a specialist in mental health care.

Key Messages

- *Female adult acne is of two types—(1) persistent acne, and (2) late-onset acne*
- *Acne relapse was a significant determinant of absenteeism/productivity loss, independently of acne severity and other variables.*

ARTICLE 81

The Mental Health Burden in Acne Vulgaris and Rosacea: An Analysis of the US National Inpatient Sample

Singam V, Rastogi S, Patel KR, et al. The mental health burden in acne vulgaris and rosacea: An analysis of the US National Inpatient Sample.
Clin Exp Dermatol. 2019.

Abstract

This study determines the mental health (MH) disorders and cost burden associated with acne and rosacea. Both acne and rosacea were associated with higher risk of mood, anxiety, impulse control and personality disorders. In particular, there were increased numbers of hospital admissions secondary to a primary MH disorder with coexistent acne/rosacea. MH comorbidities were associated with considerable excess costs among inpatients with acne or rosacea.

COMMENT

As one of the most prevalent inflammatory skin diseases, acne and rosacea are correlated with important psychosocial distress. Acne affects adolescents and young adults mainly, while rosacea is more prevalent in adults >30 years of age. Acne is associated with impaired quality of life secondary to anxiety and depression, decreased self-esteem and increased social phobia. Rosacea is associated with lower quality of life, enhanced feelings of stigma and greater levels of social anxiety owing to enhanced propensity to blush or even fear of blushing in social circumstances. This study is a retrospective study with stratified representative sample of approximately 20% of all hospitalizations in the USA. The databases were searched for a primary and secondary diagnosis of acne or rosacea using the International Classification of Diseases, Ninth Revision, Clinical Modification (ICD-9-CM) codes 706.1 and 695.3, respectively. Acne inpatients were much younger, less likely to be female, and more likely to be white/ethnic. Similarly, rosacea patients were much more likely to be male and white/ethnic, but were much older and more likely to be insured. Acne and rosacea were both associated with primary admission for depression, schizophrenia, alcohol-related disorders, developmental disorders and impulse control disorders. Acne was also associated with admission for anxiety disorders, adjustment disorders, personality disorders, substance use disorders and attention deficit disorder/attention deficit hyperactivity disorder (ADD/ADHD). Acne was not associated with suicidal hospitalization, and rosacea was inversely associated to suicidal hospitalization. Both acne and rosacea were connected in the USA with considerably higher hospital expenses and secondary care expenses for MH illnesses. A complex interaction of cutaneous and gut microbiome has been proposed to have an impact on acne severity and potentially influence systemic inflammation, oxidative stress, glycemic control and ultimately MH symptoms. Different medications, including corticosteroids and lithium, for medical and MH disorders may cause acne vulgaris and acneiform eruptions. Thus, the association of acne and rosacea with MH disorders may be secondary to medications.

Key Messages

- Acne and rosacea were associated with increased hospitalization for multiple MH, which, in turn, were associated with excess costs of care
- Clinicians should consider increased screening for MH disorders in patients with acne or rosacea, and incorporate MH disorders into therapeutic decision-making.

ARTICLE 82

The Therapeutic Effect of Tanshinone IIA on *Propionibacterium acnes*-induced Inflammation In Vitro

Li Y, Zhou Y. The therapeutic effect of tanshinone IIA on *Propionibacterium acnes*-induced inflammation in vitro.
Dermatol Ther. 2018;31(6):e12716.

Abstract

Present study evaluates the antibacterial activity of tanshinone IIA. Its effect on IL-1β, IL-8, and TNF-α expression was studied, and TLR2, NF-κB and intercellular cell adhesion molecule-1 (ICAM-1) protein level induced by *Propionibacterium acnes* in THP-1 cells were also assessed. The expression of inflammatory cytokines and TLR2, NF-κB, ICAM-1 protein levels were inhibited by Tanshinone IIA, thereby suppressing *P. acnes*-induced inflammation by blockade of TLR2/NF-κB signaling pathway.

COMMENT

Propionibacterium acnes plays a contributory role in the inflammatory lesions of acne by inducing mononuclear cells to produce inflammatory cytokines. Tanshinone IIA is a fat-soluble compound derived from Danshen and is known to play an important role in anti-inflammatory activity. The therapeutic effect and potential mechanisms of tanshinone IIA in *P. acnes*-induced inflammation was studied in this trial. Tanshinone IIA has been obtained from Salvia miltiorrhiza varvar. alba roots and purified. *Propionibacterium acnes* strain (ATCC 6919) was purchased from China Center of Industrial Culture Collection (CICC) and cultured. Human monocytic leukemia cell line THP-1 cell was obtained from the American Type Culture Collection (ATCC Manassas, VA, USA) and the cells were cultured.

For enzyme-linked immunosorbent assay (ELISA), THP-1 cells (1×10^5 cells/mL) were treated with metronidazole or concentrations of tanshinone IIA (0.05, 0.5 and 5 µM) and stimulated with living *P. acnes* (10^7 colony forming unit [CFU]/mL) for 24 hours. For quantitative real-time PCR (qRT-PCR), THP-1 cells (1×10^6 cells/mL) were treated with metronidazole or concentrations of tanshinone IIA (0.05, 0.5, 5 µM) and incubated with living *P. acnes* (10^7 CFU/mL) for 6 hours. For Western blot, THP-1 cells (5×10^5 cells/mL) were seeded into a tissue culture dish, treated with metronidazole or 0.05, 0.5 and 5 µM tanshinone IIA and then incubated with living *P. acnes* (10^7 CFU/mL) for 6 hours. MTT assay was used to detected cell viability of THP-1 cell.

They found that the cell viability exceeded 90% after even treatment with 5 µM tanshinone IIA and even the concentration range of tanshinone IIA used in THP-1 cells to evaluate their anti-inflammation against *P. acnes*-induced acne was safe and non-toxic. According to the rules of the Clinical and

Laboratory Standards Institute (Girmenia, Pizzarelli, D'Antonio, Cristini & Martino, 2003; Shungu, Weinberg & Cerami, 1985), the antibacterial activity of tanshinone IIA was evaluated using a broth microdilution technique. Human IL-1β, IL-8 and TNF-α ELISA kits (R&D Systems, Minneapolis, USA) were used to determine the concentration of IL-1β, IL-8 and TNF-α in the supernatants of cultured cells post treatment with metronidazole or tanshinone IIA for 24 hours. TRIzol reagent (Invitrogen, Carlsbad, CA) was used to isolate the total RNA from the THP-1 cells. Results showed that the production of IL-1β, IL-8 and TNF-α was increased remarkably in the *P. acnes*-treated cells, and tanshinone IIA (0.5 µM, 5 µM) significantly inhibited this response. mRNA expression of IL-1β, IL-8 and TNF-α in THP-1 cells infected with *P. acnes* was also markedly upregulated compared with control, after treatment with tanshinone IIA (0.5 µM, 5 µM), the mRNA expression of IL-1β, IL-8 and TNF-α was significantly down-regulated. Thus, the effect of tanshinone IIA on the expression of IL-8, IL-1β, and TNF-α in THP-1 cells, and found that tanshinone IIA suppressed the expression of inflammatory cytokines induced by *P. acnes* in THP-1 cells.

To know if tanshinone IIA suppresses the inflammation induced by *P. acnes* via TLR2/NF-κB signaling pathway, western blot was used to measure the TLR2, NF-κB, and ICAM-1 protein level. Results showed that the protein level of TLR2, NF-κB, and ICAM-1 was rapidly induced by *P. acnes* infection, and after treatment with various doses of tanshinone IIA, the TLR2, NF-κB, and ICAM-1 expression level was reduced remarkably. So, TLR2/NFκB signaling pathway and its downstream factor ICAM-1 was activated after infection of *P. acnes*, treatment with tanshinone IIA could inhibit the expression of TLR2, NF-κB, and ICAM-1. These results further confirmed our hypothesis that tanshinone IIA had anti-inflammation function via activating the TLR2/NF-κB pathway in THP-1 cells.

Key Message

- Tanshinone IIA inhibited *P. acnes* growth and the inflammatory cytokines by blockade of TLR2/NF-κB signaling pathway.

ARTICLE 83

Anti-acne Properties of Hydrophobic Fraction of Red Ginseng (Panax Ginseng C.A. Meyer) and its Active Components

Hou JH, Shin H, Jang KH, et al. Anti-acne properties of hydrophobic fraction of red ginseng (panax ginseng C.A. Meyer) and its active components.
Phytother Res. 2019;33(3):584-90.

Abstract

Antibiotics form a mainstay in acne management alongside retinoids. The study was done to identify the antimicrobial effects of red ginseng (panax ginseng C.A. Meyer) and to determine its potential efficacy in comparison with existing antibacterial substances. Twenty subjects with acne were treated with 3 mg/g of Red ginseng ethanol extract (RGEF) for 4 weeks, oxidized sebum contents and redness of the skin were reduced and symptoms improved especially in early and middle stages of acne. The hydrophobic fraction in RGEF showed better antimicrobial activity against *Propionibacterium acnes*.

COMMENT

Topical antibacterial agents are well validated in acne management. However, here authors have tried a natural medicine, ginseng (Panax ginseng C.A. Meyer) known to improve immunity, enhances blood flow, photoprotections and antioxidant activity due to saponin component. Another component polyacetylene is found to have antibacterial and anti-inflammatory role. In this study, active ingredients from red ginseng were studied in twenty subjects with mild-to-moderate acne—3 mg/g of Red ginseng ethanol extract (RGEF) was applied twice daily for 4 weeks, followed up at 0, 2 and 4 weeks; oil contents, oxidized sebum contents and redness of skin were measured. RGEF were prepared as an extraction with 70% alcohol at 70° C for 8 hours and a hydrophobic fraction were obtained. The anti-acne activity was analyzed by disc diffusion method. Antimicrobial spectrum was determined by comparing with triclosan and skin safety test were also performed.

RGEF showed better antibacterial property in comparison with benzoyl peroxide at 12.5 mg/mL and azelaic acid with minimum inhibitory concentration 156.3 µg/mL. Reversed silica semipreparative MPLC was done to find the active ingredients of RGEF; Panaxydol and Panaxynol were found to be the active ingredients having antibacterial activities against *Propionibacterium acnes*. The antimicrobial range of RGEF with triclosan as control, showed activity against gram-positive strains (*Bacillus subtilis, S. aureus, S. mutans*) and gram-negative and anaerobic *F. nucleatum*. Against *P. acnes*, antimicrobial activity was estimated to be 63.6%.

On clinical grounds, oil contents were significantly decreased after 2 (54.700 ± 29.439 µg/cm^2) and 4 weeks (35.800 ± 22.860 µg/cm^2) (<0.05) after application, oxidized sebum contents were at 2 and 4 weeks white/black heads, papules decreased at 2 and 4 weeks, also skin redness statistically decreased at 2 weeks (10.818 ± 2.584) and 4 weeks (10.773 ± 2.529) (<0.025). However, no significant improvements with respect to nodules were noted.

Hence, this study showed promising results of RGEF in mild-to-moderate acne. With antibacterial effect, decrease in oil and sebum content was attributed to saponins acting as surfactants.

> **Key Messages**
> - Red ginseng extract is a good option antimicrobial agent in acne care armamentarium
> - It has antibacterial and anti-inflammatory effects on acne, panaxynol acts as key antimicrobial constituent.

ARTICLE 84

Mechanistic Insight into the Activity of a Sulfone Compound Dapsone on *Propionibacterium* (Newly Reclassified as *Cutibacterium*) Acnes–mediated Cytokine Production

Geyfman M, Debabov D, Poloso N, et al. Mechanistic insight into the activity of a sulfone compound dapsone on *Propionibacterium* (newly reclassified as *Cutibacterium*) *acnes*–mediated cytokine production.
Experiment Dermatol. 2019;28(2):190-7.

Abstract

To achieve the best clinical outcome in acne, understanding of the mechanism of action of drug is critical to gain mechanistic insight into the anti-inflammatory activity of dapsone in "*Cutibacterium*" (*Propionibacterium acnes*) driven inflammation, authors have used two human *in vitro* models—primary human neonatal epidermal keratinocytes and human monocytes (THP-1). The production of interleukin (IL)-1α and IL-8 in human epidermal keratinocytes and IL-1β, IL-6, IL-8 and tumor necrosis factor-α in THP-1 cells in response to *P. acnes* was suppressed by Dapsone. THP-1 cell *in vitro* model showed that IL1β and CASP-1 were regulated by dapsone independently of NFκB activity at transcriptional and post-transcriptional levels, respectively.

COMMENT

Dapsone has antimicrobial activity and anti-inflammatory properties; however, the mechanism of dapsone on *Propionibacterium acnes*-associated inflammation is poorly understood. The authors used two *in vitro* models, primary human neonatal epidermal keratinocytes, HEKn, as a model of an early proinflammatory player in acne pathogenesis and a human myeloid monocytic cell line, THP-1, as a model of a professional innate immunity component, to investigate whether dapsone affects proinflammatory cytokine production in response to *P. acnes*. An Enzyme-Linked Immunosorbent Assay Method (ELISA) was done to determine cytokine concentrations, NF-κB activation, CASP-1 and pro- and cleaved forms of IL-1β in response to *P. acnes* in the presence of dapsone in THP-1 cells were also measured.

Phosphate buffered saline diluted viable *P. acnes* (ATCC 6919) were cocultured with HEKn cells at 50:1 (bacteria:keratinocytes) ratio together with 0 μg/mL, 0.4 μg/mL, 4 μg/mL and 40 μg/mL concentrations of dapsone, in addition, to control wells without *P. acnes*. In HEKn cells, IL-1α and IL-8 showed a 40% significant induction with the addition of *P. acnes*. Dapsone significantly reduced the IL-1α and IL-8 concentration in the media. Dapsone at a concentration of 40 μg/mL decreased the IL8 concentration below the level seen in unstimulated cells not treated with dapsone.

Coincubated undifferentiated human leukemia-derived monocytes, THP-1 (ATCC ATCC#TIB-202), with *P. acnes* (ATCC 6919) at 20:1 (bacteria: monocyte) ratio together with 0 μg/mL, 0.4 μg/mL, 4 μg/mL and 40 μg/mL concentrations of dapsone showed greater than 60% induction of IL-1β, IL-6, IL-8 and TNF-α levels in a dose-dependent manner. But, Dapsone did not lead to the reduction of NF-κB activity in THP-1 cells in response to *P. acnes*; however, it reduced inflammasomes proteins Pro- and Cleaved IL-1β and CASP-1 in a dose-dependent way in response to *P. acnes* when incubated with THP-1 cells. mRNA levels of IL-1β and its downstream target genes *IL-8* and *TNF-α* genes were also reduced 4-, 3- and 2.7-fold, respectively, with the addition of dapsone but not level of CASP-1 (Casp-1 mRNA is not affected by dapsone). Thus, the authors comment that IL-1β and its downstream cytokine genes will be regulated at a transcriptional level, while CASP-1 is regulated post-transcriptionally or post-translationally. Dapsone topically also as an antimicrobial and anti-inflammatory agent is capable of targeting inflammation in acne vulgaris pathogenesis in both epithelial and immune cells.

In this study, the mechanistic explanation for these observations isn't explained as to how IL-1β is regulated by dapsone in the absence of NFκ; CASP-1 mRNA level is not altered by dapsone, while the protein level is reduced and mechanism governing the anti-inflammatory activity of dapsone in keratinocytes. IL-1β is hypothesized by authors as an upstream regulator, tuning IL-6, TNF-α, and IL-8 and potentially other downstream cytokine genes.

Key Messages

- Dapsone can reduce P. acnes-mediated proinflammatory cytokine secretion in both keratinocyte and monocytic cell cultures
- Dapsone reduces the expression of CASP-1, as well as the substrate of active CASP-1 itself, pro-IL-1β, in response to P. acnes thus decreasing the ultimate output of inflammasome machinery–cleaved IL-1β.

ARTICLE 85

Lipidomics Reveals Skin Surface Lipid Abnormity in Male Youth Acne

Zhou M, Gan Y, He C, et al. Lipidomics reveals skin surface lipid abnormity in male youth acne.
Br J Dermatol. 2018;179(3):732-40.

Abstract

Skin surface lipids (SSL) have a main role in the initiation of the acne lesions. In this study, analytical technique, Ultra-performance liquid chromatography-quadrupole time-of-flight mass spectrometry (UPLC-QTOF-MS), was used to investigate the SSL variations of lipid main classes, subclasses and individual species in 70 subjects (35 acne patients and 35 controls). Significantly increased levels of glycerophospholipids (GP), fatty acyls (FA) and sterol lipids (ST) and decreased levels of prenol lipids (PR) and saccharolipids (SL) were found in acne patients; 18 subclasses significantly varied; phosphatidylserines (PS) were the majority of differentiating lipid species found. Also, reduction of ceramides chain length and increase in unsaturated free fatty acids, contributed to an altered lipid organization and decreased skin barrier function in acne patients.

COMMENT

Acne etiopathogenesis is primarily due to skin surface lipid (SSL) alterations, hormone levels, bacterial infection and inflammatory reaction. In this prospective, comparative study a powerful analytical technique, ultra-performance liquid chromatography-quadrupole time of flight-mass spectrometry (UPLC-QTOF-MS), has been used to investigate the SSL variations of lipid main classes, subclasses and individual species.

Seventy subjects (35 acne patients, age 22.3 ± 2.0 and 35 controls, age 23.5 ± 1.4) were recruited, clinically acne graded, sampling of all severe acne patients lesional skin was done by placing a Sebutape® test strip. The SSL on Sebutape® were collected by a modified Bligh and Dyer method, and the lipid extract was dried using low-temperature concentrator SpeedVac SPD131P; redissolved in a reagent mixture and analyzed in UPLC-QTOF-MS. High-resolution mass measurements were performed with a Waters Xevo G2-XS QTOF-MS. Data extraction and analysis were performed by Waters Progenesis QI 2.0. A comparison with the LIPID MAPS (http://www.lipidmaps.org/) Structure Database (LMSD) was performed to identify the compound ID of lipid composition of each sample.

Eight-hundred and seventy-four lipids were identified and they were all classified into eight assigned main classes. In acne patients, significant increased ($p < 0.05$) levels of three main classes [fatty acyls (FA), glycerophospholipids (GP) and sterol lipids (ST)] and significant decreased ($p < 0.05$)

levels of two main classes [prenol lipids (PR) and saccharolipids (SL)] were found, whereas there was no significant change of the relative amount of other three main classes [glycerolipids (GL), sphingolipids (SP) and polyketides (PK)]; 18 subclasses significantly varied ($p < 0.05$) and shared the same changing trends of their belonging main classes. SSL sampled from acne patients had significantly higher levels of phosphatidylserines (PS). PS exposure might be an important event during inflammation and the following cell apoptosis of acne lesions.

Content comparison of several well-known individual lipid species had also been analyzed; cholesterol, wax esters and squalene-related compounds (triterpenes) were at higher levels of SSL in acne patients than that of controls, whereas linoleic acid (and its precursor) was at lower level in acne patients.

Increased TEWL values were determined in acne patients compared to that of controls, indicating that the skin barrier was impaired in acne patients (acne patients—16.56 ± 4.31 and controls—12.05 ± 2.58). A high affinity between skin barrier function with the chain length of free fatty acids (FFAs) and Ceramides (Cers), and the relative amount of unsaturated and saturated FFAs was noted. In acne patients, significant increased levels of unsaturated FFAs and decreased levels of saturated FFAs were monitored compared to that of controls, whereas there was no significant change in average FFA chain length in two groups; a significant decrease of average Cer chain length in acne patients compared with controls. Thus, the reduction of Cers chain length and increase in unsaturated FFAs, contribute to an altered lipid organization and decreased skin barrier function in acne.

Key Messages

- Variations of SSL composition are the main factors in the induction of acne inflammation and in the following cell apoptosis
- Reduction of ceramides chain length and increase in unsaturated free fatty acids, contributed to an altered lipid organization and decreased skin barrier function in acne patients.

ARTICLE 86

Acne Vulgaris Severity Graded by In Vivo Reflectance Confocal Microscopy and Optical Coherence Tomography

Fuchs CS, Andersen AJ, Ardigo M, et al. Acne vulgaris severity graded by in vivo reflectance confocal microscopy and optical coherence tomography.
Lasers Surg Med. 2019;51(1):104-13.

Abstract

The study throws light on morphological characteristics of acne that may be associated with clinical acne severity through combined use of in vivo reflectance confocal microscopy (RCM) and optical coherence tomography (OCT). A total of 108 RCM image blocks and 54 OCT scans were analyzed; lesional, perilesional and lesion-free skin areas were included. Acne lesions, infundibular regions of follicles and inflammation degree were compared in acne patients and healthy participants; distinctive follicle infundibulum characteristics and inflammation were associated with acne severity.

COMMENT

In vivo reflectance confocal microscopy (RCM) and optical coherence tomography (OCT) are imaging techniques that offer visualization of epidermis and upper dermis; while dynamic OCT (D-OCT) is a software tool that detects changes in speckle variance validated for imaging of cutaneous blood flow. Authors have made an effort to identify morphological characteristics of acne that may be associated with clinical acne severity by means of combining these three modalities. In acne patients, two facial skin areas were examined with RCM (Vivascope Multilaser 15001, Caliber ID Inc., Rochester, NY – 785 nm mode) and OCT (OCT system (VivoSight 1 Dx, Michelson Diagnostics Ltd., Kent, UK); lesional skin-areas with comedones, papules, and/or pustules and perilesional skin areas more than 500 mm away from an acne lesion. Anatomical locations represented cheeks (n = 23 sites) and forehead (n = 4 sites). Further, a lesion-free site was evaluated in RCM images of preauricular skin of 10 patients. In healthy participants also in each area cheek (n = 7 sites) and preauricular region (n = 7 sites) 6 × 6 mm RCM and OCT scans were performed.

A total of 21 participants (12 men, 9 women aged 18–44, mean 25 years) were included; 14 patients with a clinical diagnosis of acne vulgaris (IGA 1–3) and 7 healthy participants (IGA 0). About 80 RCM Vivablocks 1 each from acne patients, 28 RCM Vivablocks 1 each from healthy participants, 40 OCT scans from acne patients, and 14 OCT scans from healthy participants were evaluated. Outcome measures and results were—(i) follicular infundibulum diameter: Comedones: (n = 38) diameter smaller in closed comedones (mean 192 ± 36 mm) compared to open comedones (mean 376 ± 115 mm, p <0.001) with amorphous gray material with white dots, Papule (n = 7) -infundibular diameter was 1,153 ± 742 mm with granular, light gray debris in RCM; Pustules - n = 13, circular structures with enlarged infundibulum. In OCT scans, closed comedones were well defined, had no epidermal opening, open comedones had dilated infundibulum protruding through the epidermis, papules were well-defined, dark gray, dome-shaped structures located in the deeper epidermal and papillary dermis with an either intact or thin and uneven epidermal surface (ii) morphological description of infundibular border (IGA 0, n = 131, IGA 1-3, n = 343); Hair follicles appeared coarse, oblique to vertical structures, similar in acne patients and in controls. (iii) morphological description of infundibular content; With mean infundibulum diameter of 109 mm for all follicles, but the diameter of follicles with content was increased by 25 mm (p = 0.005) and diameter of follicles in patients with IGA 3 was larger compared to follicles of IGA 0, IGA 1 and IGA 2 patients (p <0.029). Hyperreflective border, larger diameters and with amorphous and/or keratotic content represented microcomedones (iv) density of inflammatory cells increased in epidermis in IGA 3 patients compared to IGA 2 (p = 0.001); and (v) blood flow assessments: Mean blood flow was 0.210 AU (arbitrary units), SD 0.048 in controls; 0.184 AU (SD 0.041) in IGA 1 patients; 0.228 AU (SD 0.072) in IGA 2 patients; and 0.249 AU (SD 0.063) in IGA 3 patients.

Thus, patients with more severe acne had follicles with enlarged infundibulum diameter, hyperkeratotic follicular borders and hyperreflective keratinous content, and increased number of inflammatory cells and blood flow in perilesional and lesion-free skin areas. Microcomedones were common in acne patients and the density of microcomedones positively associated with acne severity.

Drawbacks of the study were unexpected result that IGA 2 patients had lower epidermal inflammation and less hyperkeratotic follicular borders than IGA 1 patients with lower blood flow the IGA 1 group which may be due to smaller sample size.

To conclude, combining RCM and OCT for acne imaging gives synergistic effect; RCM gives morphological information on cellular level and a horizontal perspective of hair follicles and hair follicle content to a depth of 200 mm which can be used to describe infundibular diameter, superficial inflammatory burden, superficial infundibular keratinous lining and microcomedones, whereas OCT qualitatively identifies deeper located acne lesions and visualizes blood flow giving functional information.

Key Messages

- Acne severity was positively associated with large follicular infundibulum diameter, white hyperkeratotic follicle border, white hyperreflective content inside follicles, and microcomedones visualized by RCM
- Inflammation degree in perilesional and lesion-free acne skin was correlated with acne severity, using density of inflammatory cells and blood flow as surrogate markers.

ARTICLE 87

Vitamin D Levels in Acne Vulgaris Patients Treated with Oral Isotretinoin

El-Hamd MA, El Taieb MA, Ibrahim HM, et al. Vitamin D levels in acne vulgaris patients treated with oral isotretinoin. *J Cosmet Dermatol.* 2019;18(1):16-20.

Abstract

The article aims to study role of Vitamin D in acne vulgaris (AV). Ninety patients with AV and 60 age-sex matched healthy subject as controls were recruited. Serum levels of 25 hydroxy vitamin D (25-OH-Vit D) in both were estimated and found to be significantly higher in patients with AV than healthy controls ($p = 0.001$) with a significant inverse relation between level of 25-OH-Vit D and severity of AV before treatment ($p = 0.001$). Serum levels of 25-OH-Vit D were significantly increased after isotretinoin treatment ($p = 0.001$). Thus, vitamin D may play a potential role in pathogenesis of AV or AV may have a negative effect on vitamin D synthesis.

COMMENT

Vitamin D is known to regulate the immune system and the proliferation and differentiation of keratinocytes and sebocytes. In vitro, SZ95 sebocytes have expressed vitamin D receptor, vitamin D-25-hydroxylase, 25 hydroxy vitamin D D-1alphahydroxylase, and 1,25-dihydroxyvitamin D-24-hydroxylase and incubation of SZ95 sebocytes with 1,25 (OH)2 D3 leads to a dose-dependent modulation of cell proliferation, cell cycle regulation, lipid content, and IL-6 and IL-8 secretion (antioxidant and anticomedogenic properties). Vitamin D deficiency may therefore lead to acne vulgaris (AV)pathogenesis. Authors conducted a case-control study on 90 patients with moderate to very severe AV and 60 age-sex matched healthy subjects as controls. Global acne grading system (GAGS) was used to group patients into moderate, severe, and very severe cases. Body mass index (BMI) was calculated for both and were treated with isotretinoin (0.75 mg/kg/day) for a period of 3 months. Ten milliliters of venous blood was aseptically drawn from each subject, one part sent for full blood picture, fasting lipids, and liver function tests (done before and monthly during the treatment period to assess any side effect of treatment) and second was used for vitamin D level measurement. Two milliliters of blood was allowed to clot and then centrifuged at 1,000 g for 15 minutes, and the serum separated for quantitative determination of 25 hydroxy vitamin D using commercial automated chemiluminescent microparticle immunoassay (Architect, Abbott Diagnostics, New Cairo, Egypt).

About 90 patients (27 males and 63 females) and 60 age-sex matched healthy control group (15 males and 45 females) were recruited. No significant differences were found between patients and controls regarding age (20.73 ± 3.32 vs. 23.80 ± 7.37 years) and BMI (23.26 ± 4.18 vs. 22.22 ± 5.39), respectively (p >0.05). Serum levels of 25-OH-Vit D were significantly lower in patients with AV than the control group (p = 0.001). According to GAGS, moderate AV 66 (73.7%) patients, severe 18 (20%) patients, and very severe 6 (6.7%) patients were found. 25-OH-Vit D level was 18.54 ± 8.30 ng/mL in patients with moderate acne, was 14.56 ± 3.98 ng/mL, and 11.32 ± 6.45 ng/mL in severe and very severe acne. In comparison, 25-OH-Vit D level in the control group was 44.83 ± 11.91 ng/mL. There was a significant inverse relation between level of 25-OH-Vit D and severity of AV before treatment (p = 0.001) and also, serum level of 25-OH-Vit D before and after isotretinoin treatment in patients with AV (p = 0.001). No important differences between patients with AV before and 3 months after isotretinoin therapy in full blood images, serum lipids and liver enzymes. In this study, significant low serum levels of 25-OH-Vit D in AV patients compared with controls and inversely related with acne severity suggesting that there is a connection between low vitamin D and acne. This study showed a significant increase in serum levels of 25-OH-Vit D after 3 months of treatments with oral isotretinoin in patients with AV.

Key Message

- Levels of vitamin D are inversely correlated with acne vulgaris severity. Vitamin D may play a potential role in acne vulgaris or acne vulgaris negatively affects vitamin D synthesis.

ARTICLE 88

The Effect of Milk Consumption on Acne: A Meta-analysis of Observational Studies

Dai R, Hua W, Chen W, et al. The effect of milk consumption on acne: A meta-analysis of observational studies.
J Eur Acad Dermatol Venereol. 2018;32(12):2244-53.

Abstract

The article is a compendium of comprehensive databases search of Pubmed, Embase, Medline and Cochrane Library, 4 cohort studies and 9 case-control or cross-sectional studies, including a total of 71,819 participants. Pooled odds ratio (OR) with its 95% confidence interval (CI) using a random-effects model was done with subgroup analyses on acne severity, milk forms and milk intake levels. Compared with nonconsumers, the pooled OR was 1.16 (95% CI 1.09–1.24) for overall milk consumers, and 1.17 (95% CI 1.10–1.24) in cohort studies, and 1.16 (95% CI 1.09–1.24) in case-control or cross-sectional studies. A stronger association in skim milk consumers (OR = 1.24, 95% CI 1.13–1.37) than in low-fat consumers (OR = 1.14, 95% CI 1.08–1.22) and full-fat consumers (OR = 1.13, 95% CI 1.05–1.21) was obtained. This meta-analysis provides evidence of a positive association between milk consumption and acne risk.

COMMENT

A meta-analysis of observational studies in accordance with the MOOSE published on milk consumption and acne was done. Acne was categorized as noninflammatory (mild), inflammatory and acne with both lesions (moderate-to-severe one) and milk products were divided into three subtypes—full-fat or whole milk, low-fat milk and skim milk. Regarding frequency of intake—high intake—consuming more than one glass of milk per day and the group with medium intake as drinking one glass of milk per day or less. The quality of each included study was assessed using the Newcastle-Ottawa Scale (NOS).

A total of 212 articles were retrieved, 181 articles were screened, 26 articles were considered of interest and assessed. About 4 cohort studies, 5 case-control and 4 cross-sectional studies were included. Number of the participants included in individual studies ranged from n=60 to n = 47,355 (M = 5524, SD = 12,227) and a total of 10,968 (26%) males; overall OR, based on 4 cohort and 10 case-control or cross-sectional studies, was 1.16 (95% CI 1.09–1.24). The pooled OR was 1.17 (95% CI 1.10–1.24) for cohort studies, and 1.16 (95% CI 1.09–1.24) for case-control or cross-sectional studies separately indicating a significant increase of acne incidence in milk drinkers with no substantial heterogeneity. A significant difference was found between milk consumption and moderate-to-severe acne (OR 1.18, 95% CI 1.01–1.37) with no obvious heterogeneity. Regarding association between intake of types of milk and acne dose-risk relationship exists; Pooled ORs were 1.13 (95% CI 1.05–1.21) for full-fat milk, 1.14 (95% CI 1.08–1.22) for low-fat milk and 1.24 (95% CI 1.13–1.37) for skim milk and between acne and milk intake level ORs were 1.08 (95% CI 1.00–1.17) for medium intake of milk and 1.12 (95% CI 1.01–1.24) for high intake of milk, respectively. In the present meta-analysis, milk intake was associated with an increased risk of acne; moderate-to-severe acne was linked to milk consumption while the mild one showed no association.

Authors conclude that milk played a role in the inflammatory process of acne and total whey protein intake from milk contributes to acne pathogenesis. Milk contains androgens, 5α-reduced steroids and other nonsteroidal growth factors, which increase IGF-1 level. IGF-1, milk-derived BCAAs and protein α-lactalbumin then active mTORC1; cause sebaceous lipogenesis, increases the synthesis of androgens - its activity and receptor signaling causing acne in the end.

Limitations of the study were less cohort studies, ambiguous diagnostic criteria for acne and unclear data on pasteurization status of milk and dairy products. A significant heterogeneity of the analysis for case-control or cross-sectional studies was also found with publication bias in the subgroup analysis. Further studies are needed to understand effect of milk processing, pasteurization status and microRNA bioavailability on acne pathogenesis.

> **Key Messages**
> - Hormonal contents, a-lactalbumin and BCAAs of milk may be responsible for the development of acne
> - Diet recommendation for acne prevention should consider limiting intake of milk.

ARTICLE 89

Acne and Nutrition: Hypotheses, Myths and Facts

Claudel JP, Auffret N, Leccia MT, et al. Acne and nutrition: Hypotheses, myths and facts.
J Eur Acad Dermatol Venereol. 2018;32(10):1631-7.

Abstract

Air pollution, aggressive skin care products, medication, mechanical, hormonal, family factors and, more recently, lifestyle and stress, have been implicated in acne, though sufficient evidence for direct causation is still lacking. The article focusses on role of nutritional elements and behavior like excessive intake of dairy products and hyperglycemic food, modern lifestyle nutrition, obesity and eating disorders in acne.

COMMENT

The review intends to provide an overview on the overall role of nutrition and associated factors in acne, sources of literature include PubMed searched randomized studies and level C (case-control or cohort studies) data. Articles on dairy products, hyperglycemic food and whey proteins have been found to be associated with acne trigger.

Nutrition factors potentially impacting on acne—(i) Dairy products: They influence acne through hormonal mediators by increasing plasma insulin-like growth factor (IGF)-1 levels, especially skimmed milk was associated with higher plasma IGF-1 levels and was more acnegenic; also, industrial cow's milk had higher anabolic steroids and other growth factors, such as progestin testosterone precursors which triggers acne; (ii) Whey proteins: Found in protein supplements are potent inducers of glucose-dependent insulinotropic polypeptides stimulating insulin secretion of pancreatic β-cells and acne causation; (iii) Hyperglycemic food favors unregulated tissue growth including follicle by simultaneously elevating the free IGF-1 level and reducing levels of IGF binding protein 3; (iv) Alcohol is nutritive for Cutibacterium acnes, increases testosterone levels, suppresses immune system on chronic consumption thereby, increases cytokine release which may influence acne; (v) Tea, coffee and chocolate: No data exists about the potential relationship between the consumption of caffeine, tea and the onset or worsening of acne, but chocolate bars containing sugar and milk may be acnegenic; (vi) Salt: No sufficient evidence that a high sodium chloride diet triggers acne, but few studies have reported increased acne in high sodium diet consumers; (vii) Associated factors: Uncontrolled food intake, obesity and eating disorders (anorexia nervosa and bulimia nervosa) have also been attributed.

Nutrients which are potentially beneficial in acne—fish products with low n-3 to n-6 polyunsaturated fatty acids (PUFA), low glycemic, lipid and transfatty acid load may help to reduce the risk of acne. Low intake of fruit or vegetables triggers acne.

Nutrition and potential targets in acne— Diet-induces changes in sebum quantity and composition, especially IGF-1 may not only induce the inflammation of acne but may also drive the process of comedogenesis. Saturated fatty acids increase the release of toll like receptor2/interleukin-1β (TLR2/IL-1β) signaling of dendritic cells, promoting Th17 cell differentiation and an increased secretion of IL-17A causes keratinocyte hyperproliferation and acne. Moreover, insulin and IGF-1, both stimulated by milk products and whey protein intake activates the PI3K-Akt pathway causing sebaceous lipogenesis. Increased Akt/mTORC1 signaling pathway enhances sebocyte survival, growth and lipogenesis, thus promoting hyperseborrhea and dysseborrhea with an exaggerated release of sebum-free fatty acids promoting inflammation.

Thus, article concludes that nutrition may potentially play a role in acne, so, daily food habits, potential family acne history, lifestyle or eating disorders should be evaluated.

Key Messages

- *Identification of potential triggers, such as dairy products, mainly skimmed milk, hyperglycemic load and the excessive intake of whey protein though have been attributed in acne causation, evidence is still insufficient*
- *Their identification may therefore allow for the better management of acne in certain patients, thus making nutrition control an additional element in the armamentarium of acne care.*

ARTICLE 90

Enhancement of Lipid Content and Inflammatory Cytokine Secretion in SZ95 Sebocytes by Palmitic Acid Suggests a Potential Link between Free Fatty Acids and Acne Aggravation

Choi CW, Kim Y, Kim JE, et al. Enhancement of lipid content and inflammatory cytokine secretion in SZ95 sebocytes by palmitic acid suggests a potential link between free fatty acids and acne aggravation.
Exp Dermatol. 2019;28(2):207-10.

Abstract

The study attempts to understand and substantiate the hypothesis that free fatty acids (FFAs) increase the production of sebum and induces inflammation in the sebaceous glands, a link exists between acne and FFAs and pave way to the development of novel treatment options for acne. Authors found that treatment of SZ95 sebocytes with exogenously applied palmitic acid (PA) induced a significant increase in intracellular lipid levels and also increased the expression and secretion of the proinflammatory cytokines in SZ95 sebocytes. Toll-like receptors had a role in inflammatory response triggered by PA.

COMMENT

Free fatty acids (FFAs) are a major component of sebum; changes in FFA affect both the synthesis of sebum and the inflammatory response in sebaceous glands. Palmitic acid (PA), a major saturated FFA, appears to play an important role in these damaging inflammation mediated effects. Exogenous FFAs may increase the production of sebum. The research tries to explore the impact of PA by ELISA, real-time PCR, petroleum red O staining, and triglyceride (TG) quantitation on the production of proinflammatory cytokines and lipogenesis. To identify the intracellular signal transduction pathway Western blotting assay was done and anti-TLR antibodies were used to investigate the role of TLRs in the inflammation induced by PA.

Treatment with PA for SZ95 sebocytes led to a substantial rise in intracellular lipid levels observed by oil red O staining and also reduced the quantity of intracellular TGs in these cells in a dose-dependent way. Thus, exogenous PA apparently increased the levels of intracellular lipids that are components of sebum. PA mediated changes in proinflammatory cytokine (IL-6 and IL-8) expression was significantly increased in dose-dependent manner on treatment of sebocytes with PA.

To understand the role of intracellular signal transduction pathway, phosphorylation levels of several key signaling molecules were done by assessing the levels of phosphorylated IκB, JNK and Akt. PA treatment increased the phosphorylation of IκB and JNK in SZ95 sebocytes in a dose-dependent manner; FFA activated NF-κB and JNK pathways in these cells but, the level of phosphorylated Akt was not changed after PA treatment.

Toll-like receptor (TLR2 and TLR4), affected PA-induced cytokine changes in SZ95 sebocytes. After pretreatment with anti-TLR2 or anti-TLR4 antibody, the cells were treated with PA, and the secretion of IL-6 and IL-8 was evaluated; Pam3CSK4 and LPS were used as a positive control. Pretreatment with an anti-TLR2 antibody significantly diminished PA-induced increase in IL-6 secretion by SZ95 sebocytes, whereas pretreatment with an anti-TLR4 antibody did not. PA-mediated secretion of IL-8 was attenuated by the pretreatment with either anti-TLR2 or anti-TLR4 antibody. Taken together, these results indicate that TLR2 and TLR4 are required during the inflammatory response activated by PA in SZ95 sebocytes.

Thus, the article concludes that FFAs induces sebaceous gland inflammation and exogenous PA significantly increases the levels of proinflammatory cytokines in SZ95 sebocytes. The article also throws light on the role of toll-like receptors (TLRs) in the molecular mechanism of PA-induced pro-inflammatory cytokine production.

Key Message
- Exogenous PA increases not only the levels of intracellular lipids that are contained in the sebum, but also production of inflammatory cytokines through TLR2 and TLR4.

ARTICLE 91

Characterization of *Cutibacterium acnes* Phylotypes in Acne and In Vivo Exploratory Evaluation of Myrtacine

Pécastaings S, Roques C, Nocera T, et al. Characterization of *Cutibacterium acnes* phylotypes in acne and in vivo exploratory evaluation of Myrtacine.
J Eur Acad Dermatol Venereol. 2018;32:15-23.

Abstract
This is a comparative study between *Cutibacterium acnes* (*C. acnes*) skin colonization in patients with mild-to-moderate acne versus healthy controls and also evaluates a Myrtacine-based cream on *C. acnes* total population and anti-bioresistant Cutibacteria in patients with acne. *Cutibacterium acnes* was not significantly different in acne versus control groups.

COMMENT

Epidemiological studies have shown a marked increase in the frequency of topical antibiotic resistance in acne subject especially to erythromycin and clindamycin with formation of biofilm as an attributable cause. Myrtacine is able to increase the bactericidal activity of antibiotics and decrease *Cutibacterium acnes* (*C. acnes*) counts even with strains resistant to erythromycin, in vitro. Total *C. acnes* load and antibiotic-resistant Cutibacterium populations, as well as *C. acnes* phylotype repartition in the skin of acne patients were evaluated in comparison with the skin of age- and sex-matched healthy controls.

60 acne patients (Global Acne Severity Scale, GEA grades 2-3), of mean age 20 (15-30) years and 24 age- and sex- matched healthy controls were recruited with three visits—at inclusion (D0), intermediate (D28 ± 3 days) and at the end of the study (D56 ± 7 days); forehead strips samplings were performed for microbiological analysis of comedones by colony forming unit (CFU) counts of global *C. acnes* and erythromycin (EryR) or clindamycin-resistant (ClnR) populations of Cutibacterium and determination of phylotypes by MALTI-TOF. Clinical evaluations of acne patients (lesion count, porphyrin fluorescence) were performed at baseline, D28 and D56 days of twice-daily application of a Myrtacine-based cream. Finally, another microbiological sampling was realized on acne patients at D56.

About 85% had mild acne GEA grade 2, 15% moderate acne, GEA grade 3; *C. acnes* and *C. granulosum* were obtained from cultures. Mean CFU (culture) and GU (qPCR) measurements (±SD) of *C. acnes* loads showed a high total colonization by the species both in healthy controls (5.94 ± 1.01 log (CFU/strip) and 5.62 ± 0.76 log (GU/strip)) and in acne patients (6.33 ± 0.19 log (CFU/strip) and 5.62 ± 0.71 log (GU/strip)) but not statistically significant.

In 14 acne patients carrying *C. granulosum*, EryR or ClnR resistant isolates were detected in 10 patients. EryR resistant strains of *C. acnes* and *C. granulosum* were found in 56.7% of patients at baseline (n = 34/60), and 54.1% of controls (n = 13/24), without significant difference in terms of bacterial load between the two groups (5.05 ± 0.93 log CFU/strip and 4.56-0.95 log CFU/strip, respectively; $p=0.115$) while ClinR *C. acnes* and *C. granulosum* strains were detected (3-6 log CFU/strip) in acne patients (10%, n = 6/60) and controls (12.5%, n = 3/24). *C. acnes* phylotype repartition was performed on a total of 1,531 *C. acnes* isolates from healthy controls (n = 257) and acne patients (n = 1,274). A skewed distribution was associated with acne, with a 1.54-fold increase in the proportion of phylotype IA compared with healthy samples (40% vs. 26%). On the reverse, phylotypes IB-IC were 1.46-fold less frequent in acne samples (24% versus 35%). Phylotype IA was carried by 73.3% of acne patients versus 50.0% of the healthy controls ($p < 0.05$). On the contrary, a higher proportion of healthy controls carried the IB-IC phylotypes (75.0%) compared with acne patients (55.0%), Phylotype IA was dominant among EryR strains and significantly inferior in the healthy group compared with the acne group ($p < 0.05$).

Myrtacine-based cream significantly reduces the level of EryR strains of *C. acnes* in vivo, in association with a decrease of acne lesions. Total *C. acnes* load (nonsignificant change in amount of *C. acnes* (0.05 ± 0.61 log GU/strip) between D0 (5.62 ± 0.71) and D56 (5.67 ± 0.77)) and antibiotic-resistant *C. acnes* and *C. granulosum* load before and after 56 days (decreased from 4.95 ± 0.99 at D0 to 4.76 ± 1.05 at D56), production of porphyrins by *C. acnes* after 56 days of treatment (result: decreased), evolution of acne severity according to GEA scale after 29 and 56 days of treatment (highly significant ($p < 0.0001$) decrease in their severity score), evolution of retentional and inflammatory acne lesions according to ECLA grading after 29 and 56 days of treatment were performed (D56 versus D0, 37 patients (62%) showed an improvement of their ECLA score for retentional lesions, including 12 with a reduction of two grades, and 52 patients (87%) had an improvement of their ECLA score for superficial inflammatory lesions, including 19 with a reduction of two grades).

Phylotype determination of ten clones per subject and analysis of the characteristics of resistant isolates of *C. acnes* are unique to the study.

Key Messages

- Strategies to directly overcome the mechanisms of bacterial resistance and limit antibiotic use are need of the hour in acne management
- Myrtacine cream impairs the formation and/or the persistence of *C. acnes* biofilm in the pilosebaceous follicle, causing increased sensitivity of bacterial cells to the immune system and reducing erythromycin-resistant strains of Cutibacterium.

ARTICLE 92

Atrophic Scar Formation in Acne Patients involves Long-acting Immune Responses with Plasma Cells and Alteration of Sebaceous Gland

Carlavan I, Bertino B, Rivier M, et al. Atrophic scar formation in acne patients involves long-acting immune responses with plasma cells and alteration of sebaceous gland.
Br J Dermatol. 2018;179(4):906-17.

Abstract

The study was done to understand the pathophysiology of atrophic scar formation paving new therapies for the prevention of acne scarring. Large-scale gene expression profiling and immunohistochemistry analysis were performed on uninvolved skin and papules in both, scar-prone (SP) and non-scar-prone (NSP) acne patients, at different time points. Gene expression and immunohistochemistry analyzes showed a very similar immune response in 48 hour-old papules in both groups. Persistent immune response was seen in SP patients with a drastic reduction of sebaceous gland markers suggesting an irreversible destruction of sebaceous gland structures after inflammatory remodeling. Thus, the inter-relationship between duration and severity of inflammation and the alteration of sebaceous gland structures, leads to atrophic scar formation in acne.

COMMENT

In this prospective study, pathophysiological processes that occur in patients with scar-prone (SP) and non-scar-prone (NSP) acne in 21-day lesions with large-scale gene expression profiling have been researched and interpreted to define molecular and cellular pathways responsible for scarring. Patients with moderate inflammatory acne as defined by the ECLA score, 10 prone to scarring and 9 non-prone to scarring, were enrolled. Biopsies of non-lesional skin (NLS) and of inflammatory lesions less than 48 hour old, were taken on the back of scar-prone (SP) and non-scar-prone (NSP) patients. In addition, lesions less than 48 hours of age were recognized and followed for 21 days. At day 21 a biopsy was taken at this location, and designated as "evolved lesions" (SP-EL for scar-prone patients and NSP-EL for non-scar-prone patients). Additional normal skin biopsies from 10 healthy volunteers were acquired for immunohistochemistry to be compared with the uninvolved skin of patients with acne. For gene expression profiling of human sebaceous glands and epidermis, skin samples were obtained from 5 healthy individuals undergoing plastic surgery. Probes were synthesized and then hybridized on Affymetrix U133 Plus 2.0 chips (Affymetrix, Santa Clara, CA). Data analysis and identification of differentially expressed genes were done using a two-sided paired T test with Array Studio software (OmicSoft Corporation, USA). Genes with fold change |FCH| >2 and false discovery rate (FDR) <0.05 were selected. Non-Negative Matrix Factorization, NMF, was applied to cluster samples and select genes that account for the specificity of each cluster.

Profiles of gene expression of 21-day lesions developed varied between SP and NSP populations. Two major clusters emerged following unsupervised clustering of gene expression data including 48 hours old papules and non-lesional skin. 660 and 543 unique genes were differentially expressed in papules from NSP and SP patients, respectively, compared to patient-matched non-lesional skin.

Next, the gene expression profiles of evolved lesions (21 days of age) were added to the NMF clusters; there was a clear discrimination between the SP and NSP populations with respect to evolved lesions. Most heavily repressed SP-EL genes and most of these genes, such as *ELOVL3*, *AWAT1*, *FADS1* and *FADS2*, were discovered to be preferentially expressed in sebaceous glands compared to epidermis in the gene expression profile of human sebaceous glands. CD163, CD68 and EMR1 mRNA expression levels were similarly increased in papules of both populations; even higher levels in evolved lesions of the SP population. CD68 positive cells, i.e. macrophages was seen in early papules, also 21 days old ones in SP and in them recruitment of macrophages/monocytes remains elevated over time. Also, LTF lactotransferrin showed a significant >2-fold upregulation of mRNA levels in 48 hour-old papules in both NSP and SP populations, but no modulation in SP-EL.

Only in papules of both populations and in developed lesions of SP patients, a powerful T-cell infiltrate is noted. In SP-EL, the magnitude of the fold change of T cell markers, including CD4 and CD8 was greater than those observed in early papules of both populations and CD3+ cells in early papules of both populations, and in evolved lesions of the SP population was increased. But, plasma cells were involved in the immune response in evolved lesions of SP acne patients with downregulation of lipid metabolism in lesions of SP patients suggesting an alteration of sebaceous glands.

Thus, at 21 days, the gene expression profile between SP and NSP was clearly different with down-modulation of a lipid-associated gene and a strong relationship exists between severity and duration of inflammation and the development of scarring and a deep alteration of the sebaceous gland structure also lead to atrophic scar formation.

Key Message

- Inflammatory immune processes persist for at least 3 weeks in the lesions of scar-prone acne patients and so treatment regimens preventing or at least reducing the duration of inflammatory processes in scar-prone acne patients are required.

ARTICLE 93

Lesional and Circulating Levels of Interleukin-17 and 25 Hydroxy-cholecalciferol in Active Acne Vulgaris: Correlation to Disease Severity

Abd-Elmaged WM, Nada EA, Hassan MH, et al. Lesional and circulating levels of interleukin-17 and 25 hydroxy-cholecalciferol in active acne vulgaris: Correlation to disease severity.
J Cosmet Dermatol. 2019;18(2):671-6.

Abstract

This article is a cross-sectional, case-control study on 135 patients with active acne vulgaris and 150 matched controls. The aim of the study is to analyze the role of IL-17 and 25 hydroxycholecalciferol (25(OH) D3) in the pathogenesis and progression of acne vulgaris. Higher IL-17 expression levels in active acne lesions with significantly lower levels of Vitamin D3; significantly negative correlations between IL-17 and 25(OH)D3 levels (p <0.001 for both were found).

COMMENT

This case-control, hospital-based study included 135 patients with active acne vulgaris. Acne severity was graded, using Global Acne Grading Scale (GAGS). About 150 healthy volunteers, age, body mass index, and sex matched constituted the control group. Serum IL-17 and 25(OH)D3 were estimated using commercially available ELISA assay kits supplied by Chongqing Biopsies Co., Ltd, Chongqing, China (Catalog No. BEK1123 for IL-17 and BYEK1472 for 25(OH)D3). Measurements were taken using ELISA multiskan EX micro-platephotometer (STAT FAX-2100; Thermo Scientific, Palm City, FL, USA). Skin punch biopsies were taken from the acne lesion; first part homogenized using lysis buffer (Tris-HCl), pH 7.4 in ice-cold. ELISA determination of tissue 25(OH)D3 and IL-17 levels was done with Western blotting assessment of lesional IL-17 expression. The second part of the biopsy was washed with saline and fixed in 10% formaldehyde for histopathological examination.

About 135 patients had active acne (54 males and 81 females) with their mean age 21.04 ± 2.8 SD years and 150 controls (78 males and 72 female) with mean age 23.1 ± 4.6 SD years, with no significant differences between the two groups indicating age and sex matching. According to the acne severity using GAGS, patients were divided into three subgroups—mild acne (n = 45), moderate acne (n = 45), and severe acne (n = 45).

The mean serum levels of IL-17 (pg/mL), among patients and controls were 544.2 ± 477.4 SD and 42.2 ± 8.1 SD, respectively, with significantly higher levels among the patient group. There were significant increasing IL-17 serum levels with increasing acne severity. The mean lesional homogenate levels of IL17 (pg/mg tissue protein) were 0.8 ± 0.7 SD and 0.16 ± 0.02 SD in patients and controls respectively, with significantly higher levels among the patient group. There were also significant increasing IL-17 lesional homogenate levels with increasing acne severity (0.23 ± 0.08, 0.44 ± 0.08 and 1.7 ± 0.28) in patients with mild, moderate, and severe acne, respectively with higher IL-17 lesional expression levels among patients with moderate and severe acne versus mild acne and the controls when using Western blotting. Immune positivity of the membrane of epidermal degenerative cells to anti-IL17 antibody was also seen directly related to the acne severity with appearance of immune-reactive lymphocytes to anti-IL17 antibody in the dermis that increased with increased acne severity.

The mean serum levels of 25(OH)D3 (ng/mL), were 33.3 ± 9.7 SD and 51.7 ± 2.7 SD among patients and controls respectively, with significantly lower levels among the patients and with increasing acne severity; 25(OH)D3 insufficiency and deficiency in patients was 22% and 11%, respectively. The mean lesional homogenate levels of 25(OH)D3 (ng/mg tissue protein) were 0.09 ± 0.1 SD and 0.12 ± 0.05 SD among patients and controls respectively, with significantly lower levels among the patients; significant decreasing 25(OH)D3 lesional homogenate levels with increased acne severity was also noted.

There were significantly negative correlations between serum and tissue levels of IL-17 versus serum and tissue levels of 25(OH)D3 (r = −0.918, −0.724, respectively, p <0.001 for both). The present study demonstrates significant increase in the serum and tissue levels of IL-17 levels in acne patients when compared with the healthy controls, supporting the involvement of IL-17 in the inflammatory pathway of acne vulgaris with occurrence of a negative mechanistic interplay with vitamin D3 levels.

Key Message

- Deficiency of vitamin D3 with higher IL-17 in an inverse pattern has a possible role in active acne vulgaris.

ARTICLE 94

Clinical Efficacy of 0.5% Topical Mangosteen Extract in Nanoparticle Loaded Gel in Treatment of Mild-to-moderate Acne Vulgaris: A 12-Week, Split-Face, Double-blinded, Randomized, Controlled Trial

Lueangarun S, Sriviriyakul K, Tempark T, et al. Clinical efficacy of 0.5% topical mangosteen extract in nanoparticle loaded gel in treatment of mild-to-moderate acne vulgaris: A 12-week, split-face, double-blinded, randomized, controlled trial. *J Cosmet Dermatol.* 2019.

Abstract

The article is a prospective comparative study to assess the efficacy of 0.5% topical mangosteen extract in nanoparticle loaded gel (containing alpha-mangostin) compared with 1% clindamycin gel in the treatment of mild-to-moderate acne vulgaris.

COMMENT

Alpha-mangostin, active component in mangosteen (Garcinia mangostana Linn.) rind is found to have anti-skin cancer, antioxidant, anti-inflammatory, anti-allergy, antifungal, and antimicrobial properties. It also exhibits inhibitory effects to *Staphylococcus epidermidis* and *Propionibacterium acnes* (*P. acnes*) [minimum inhibitory concentration (MIC)- 0.039 mg/mL against *P. acnes*]. This action has been explored by the authors to study its effects in inflammatory acne; a comparative study using 0.5% mangostin nanoparticle loaded gel (MNLG) versus 1% clindamycin gel. The stability and irritation of MNLG was tested effectively prior to prescribing.

About 28 patients aged 18–40 years with mild-to-moderate acne vulgaris were enrolled in this double-blinded, split-face, randomized, control study. About 2.5% benzoyl peroxide cream was applied to both sides of the faces once daily for 5 minutes and washed off. Each patient was randomly treated with the mangosteen fruit rind extract on one side and 1% clindamycin on another side of the face twice daily for 12 weeks. Treatment efficacies and side effects were evaluated at 2, 4, 8 and 12 weeks.

The mean ± SD GAGs score was 15.43 ± 5.96. 24 (85.7%) females and 4 (14.3%) males were recruited with average age 25.14 ± 5.8, and the III, IV and V Fitzpatrick skin phototypes were 32%, 57%, and 11%. 0.5% (w/w) MNLG significantly reduced comedone lesions from the second week until the end of the study and the mean reduction of comedone from baseline to week 12 was 6.07 ± 5.52 to 3.04 ± 2.2 ($p < 0.001$) in MNLG-treated side accounting 66.86%, and 6.18 ± 4.7 to 2.48 ± 1.96 ($p < 0.001$) in 1% clindamycin gel-treated side accounting overall 55.33%. The average reduction of inflammatory acne counts in the MNLG and the 1% clindamycin groups was 18.32 ± 13.456.8 ± 6.34 ($p < 0.001$) (percent reduction: 67.05%) and 17.5 ± 12.878.04 ± 9.52 ($p < 0.001$) (percent reduction: 64.16%), respectively. Thus, a better improvement was seen with the grading scores of 1.33 versus 1.67, ($p = 0.004$), respectively in MNLG-treated than clindamycin-treated group.

Post-acne erythema (PAE) in both groups evaluated by biometric measurement had significant decrease in hemoglobin indices of PAE. Porphyrin severity grading, done using Wood's lamp examination at week 12 in the MNLG and the clindamycin-treated revealed significant reduction of porphyrin grading scores from the median (IQR) of 2.61 ± 0.58-1.27 ± 0.35 ($p < 0.001$) and 2.55 ± 0.6-1.25 ± 0.39 ($p < 0.001$). Side effects were minimal consisting of dryness and itching which recovered spontaneously. 0.5% (w/w) MNLG and 1% clindamycin gel did not significantly improve PIH. Thus, study concludes that MNLG is a promising adjuvant option in acne; safe and effective. But shorter period of study and small sample size are its limitations.

Key Messages

- MNLG could be a satisfactory optional phytopharmaceutical medication for acne with anti-inflammatory, antioxidant and antimicrobial properties
- For prevention of the overuse of topical antibiotics in acne patients and the avoidance of further drug-resistant bacteria such options are promising.

ARTICLE 95

The Influence of Exposome on Acne

Dréno B, Bettoli V, Araviiskaia E, et al. The influence of exposome on acne.
J Eur Acad Dermatol Venereol. 2018;32(5):812-9.

Abstract

The article provides a comprehensive review on the impact of environmental factors on acne and acne exposome. Two consensus meetings of European dermatologists and a comprehensive literature search on exposome factors triggering acne served as a basis for this review.

COMMENT

Acne exposome was defined as the sum of all environmental factors influencing the occurrence, duration and severity of acne. Exposome factors impact on the response and the frequency of relapse to treatments by interacting with the skin barrier, sebaceous gland, innate immunity, and cutaneous microbiota. Six main categories of factors are nutrition, psychological and lifestyle factors, occupational factors including cosmetics, as well as pollutants, medication and climatic factors. Review has been made from all relevant articles including epidemiological, in vitro, ex vivo and clinical studies and update from two consensus meetings of a board of European dermatologists held in July and October, 2017; and practical considerations for managing acne patients have been proposed.

Acne exposome factors

- *Nutrition*: Main food classes considered triggering acne are dairy products (especially skim milk), hyperglycemic carbohydrates, and nutritional supplements such as whey proteins containing leucine used by athletes. Acne rarely occurs in congenital deficiencies of insulin growth factor-1 (IGF-1). Oral antibiotics and probiotics (reduce systemic oxidative stress, regulate cytokines and reduce inflammatory markers) provide synergistic benefit in decreasing both inflammatory and noninflammatory acne lesions
- *Medications:* Androgenic progestins (desogestrel and 3-cetodesogestrel, levonorgestrel, lynestrenol, norgestrienone, norethisterone, norgestrel, gestodene, norgestimate and etonogestrel) and anabolic steroids trigger acne. Conversely, chlormadinone acetate, dienogest, drospirenone and norgestimate, cyproterone acetate are beneficial. Corticosteroids, halogens, isoniazid, lithium, vitamin B12, immunosuppressants and certain anticancer agents and radiotherapy cause acneiform eruptions
- *Occupational factors*: Aggressive skin care regimens and inappropriate cosmetics (comedogenic ingredients, essential oils or too greasy or oily foundations, powder make-up, aggressive skin cleansers and

soaps with pH of 8.0) may cause acne flareups by activating innate immunity and trigger inflammation
- *Mechanical factors*: Rubbing, scrubbing, the use of home devices or medical devices such as sonic brushes, dermarollers or microneedling systems flare acne (folliculitis mechanica)
- *Pollutants:* Air pollutants, industrial pollutants (Chloracne), human-dependent pollutants (Tobacco and *Cannabis*) are implicated as trigger factors
- *Climatic conditions:* Heat, humidity and intensive UVR trigger acne (acne tropicana)
- *Psychosocial and lifestyle factors*: Stress, emotion, sleep deprivation and modern lifestyle. Thus, these need to be checked at initial visit.

According to the above-described exposome factors practical considerations prior to prescription has been proposed by the authors, identify potential negative exposome factors, limit consumption of high glycemic index food in predisposed patients and food supplements containing whey proteins, decrease smoking tobacco/ *cannabis*, modifications of contraceptives and skin care regimens might be suggested. Topical antibiotics as monotherapy are not recommended. Topical retinoids combined or not with benzoyl peroxide should be prescribed in the evening. Avoid harsh washing of skin and use cleansers with a pH of 5.5 (syndet) with optimal frequency of cleansing twice a day. Moisturizers should be used in the morning and use non-comedogenic make-up and sun-protecting products with a sun-protecting factor of at least 30.

Thus, identifying the negative exposome factors and thus reducing their impact are mandatory for an adequate acne management. Skin–gut axis in patients with acne, beneficial effects of pre- and probiotics and specific regimens combining a low glycemic index diet and restricted intake of cow milk still remains to be explored by large well-designed clinical studies.

Key Message

◉ Exposome factors including nutrition, medication, occupational factors, pollutants, climatic factors, and psychosocial and lifestyle factors impact on the course and severity of acne and on treatment efficacy. Identifying and reducing the impact of exposome is important for an adequate acne disease management.

ARTICLE 96

Association of Interleukin-6 Gene Promoter Polymorphism with Acne Vulgaris and its Severity

Ragab M, Hassan EM, Elneily D, et al. Association of interleukin-6 gene promoter polymorphism with acne vulgaris and its severity.
Clin Exp Dermatol. 2019;44(6):637-42.

Abstract

Present study was undertaken to investigate the role of cytokines and mediators in acne vulgaris (AV) pathogenesis. Interleukin (IL)-6 572 polymorphism in patients with AV and its relation to patient sex and acne severity was studied in 30 patients with acne and 20 healthy controls (HCs). The Global Acne Grading System was used to assess acne severity and IL-6 572 gene promoter polymorphism was assessed using the polymerase chain reaction–restriction fragment length polymorphism (PCR–RFLP) method. A significant association of IL-6 572 variants genotypes in patients with acne (93%) compared with the HC group (45%) (p <0.001), with a higher incidence of the IL-6 572 CC polymorphism in patients with acne was found substantiating role of IL-6 gene promoter polymorphism in AV susceptibility.

COMMENT

Proinflammatory cytokines interleukin (IL)-6 has been mapped to chromosome 7p15-p21, and has five exons and four introns; three SNPs, 597 G/A (rs1800797), 572 G>C (rs1800796) and 174 G>C (rs1800795) and has also been implicated in AV. IL-6 is induced via bacterial lipopolysaccharides, second messengers, cytokines and growth factors and even keratinocytes and sebocytes; they secrete IL-6 which eventually causes trafficking of neutrophils, cytokines, proteases and free radicals production.

A prospective study on 30 patients with AV (mean age 27.60 ± 5.36 years) and 20 HCs (26.75 ± 5.25 years) was done by assessing for IL-6 polymorphism. Global Acne Grading System (GAGS) done to evaluate acne severity [Six areas evaluated (face/forehead, both cheeks, nose, chin chest and upper back): 0, no lesion detected; 1, ≥1 comedonal lesion; 2, ≥1 papule detected; 3, ≥1 pustule; and 4, ≥1 nodule]. Subscores were multiplied by a specific factor for each region, and summated, classifying acne severity as mild (1-18 points), moderate (19-30), severe (31-38) or very severe (>39). The IL-6 572 G/C polymorphism was determined using a PCR–RFLP method. Presence of one band indicated the GG genotype, two bands the CC genotype, and three bands the GC genotype.

Among patients, 3 had mild acne, 22 moderate acne and 5 severe acne. The GC + CC genotype variants were significantly more common in the patient group than in the HC group (93% vs. 45%), whereas the GG variant was more common in the HC group. The genotype frequencies for patients and HCs were, respectively, 6.7% versus 55% for GG, 46.7% versus 30% for GC, and 46.7% versus 15% for CC. Of the 30 patients, 28 had IL-6 polymorphism associations: 10 (91%) of the 11 men (35.7% of the total group) and 18 (95%) of the 19 women (64.3% of the total group) showed this polymorphism with no significant difference between men and women with regard to IL-6 genotypic variant associations (p = 1.00). Allelic frequencies showed that G allele was present in 30% of patients and 70% of HCs, whereas the percentages were reversed for the C allele, which was present in 70% and 30%, respectively. There was a significant difference between the C and G allele at the 572 position of IL-6 gene promoter in patients and HCs, with a significantly higher risk of AV development with the IL-6 572 C allele (OR = 5.44, 95% CI 2.27–13.04, p <0.001).

The incidence of the IL-6 572 C/C polymorphism was also significantly higher in patients than in HCs (46.7% vs. 15%, respectively; OR = 4.96, 95% CI 1.20–20.55, p = 0.001).

There was no significant association between the IL-6 572 genotypes and the severity of AV.

Thus, the study concluded that single nucleotide polymorphisms (SNPs) in the *IL-6* gene at position 572 may be involved in the pathogenesis of AV and no association was found between IL-6 572 variant genotypes and acne severity as measured by GAGS. However, further studies on IL-6 polymorphisms with larger sample sizes, different ethnic groups and additional SNPs are needed to verify these results.

Key Message
- The IL-6 gene promoter polymorphism might have a role in AV susceptibility but it is not related to AV severity.

ARTICLE 97

Genome-wide Meta-analysis Implicates Mediators of Hair Follicle Development and Morphogenesis in Risk for Severe Acne

Petridis C, Navarini AA, Dand N, et al. Genome-wide meta-analysis implicates mediators of hair follicle development and morphogenesis in risk for severe acne.
Nat Commun. 2018;9(1):5075.

Abstract
Acne vulgaris is a highly heritable common, chronic inflammatory disease of the skin for which five genetic risk loci have so far been identified. In this study, they identified 20 independent association signals at 15 risk loci, 12 of which have not been previously implicated in the disease. The causal variants disrupt the coding region of WNT10A and a P63 transcription factor binding site in SEMA4B. These indicate that variation affecting the structure and maintenance of the pilosebaceous unit, is a critical aspect of the genetic predisposition to severe acne.

COMMENT

Previous genome-wide association trials (GWAS) of serious acne identified five genomic loci that gave insight into the biological mechanisms underlying the pathogenesis of illness, including a potential role for TGF-β pathway elements. In the current study, they delineate the genetic susceptibility of severe acne through the identification of genetic variation at 15 genomic loci that contribute to disease risk.

This study was a meta-analysis using summary statistics from this newly performed GWAS and the previously published GWAS of severe acne in the UK population. During the anagen phase of hair development, WNT10A is heavily produced in dermal papilla within the pilosebaceous unit and is produced in the dermal condensate and neighboring follicular epithelium. The transcription factor TP63 is critically important for epidermal morphogenesis including hair follicle development and rare mutations in the *TP63* gene have also been described in monogenic ectodermal dysplasia syndromes that have substantial phenotypic overlap with ectodermal dysplasias resulting from mutation of WNT10A.

About 22% of the phenotypic variance is clarified in this research by variations across the genome. The combination of the 15 genome-wide significant loci accounts for ~3% of the phenotypic variance, indicating that there are further loci contributing to the disease susceptibility that remain undiscovered. Fine mapping and eQTL colocation of recognized association signals allowed the involvement of genes including *WNT10A*, *LGR6*, *TP63*, and *LAMC2* that developed roles in regulating hair follicle growth, morphology, and activity. The identification of this series of putative causal genes provides the basis for an appealing hypothesis that genetic susceptibility to acne results, in part, from variation in the structure and maintenance of the pilosebaceous unit that creates a follicular environment prone to bacterial colonization and resulting inflammation. This insight highlights processes that add to the growth and maintenance of hair follicles as future therapeutic objectives to complement present therapeutic systems that concentrate on inflammation suppression and colonization of bacteria.

Key Messages

- Genetic susceptibility to acne results, in part, from variation in the structure and maintenance of the pilosebaceous unit that creates a follicular environment prone to bacterial colonization and resulting inflammation
- Processes contributing to the growth and maintenance of hair follicles are prospective therapeutic objectives complementing present therapeutic systems focusing on inflammation suppression and bacterial colonization.

ARTICLE 98

Microbiological Profile of Sarecycline: A Novel Targeted Spectrum Tetracycline for the Treatment of Acne Vulgaris

Zhanel G, Critchley I, Lin LY, et al. Microbiological profile of sarecycline: a novel targeted spectrum tetracycline for the treatment of acne vulgaris.
Antimicrob Agent Chemother. 2019;63(1):e01297-18.

Abstract

The first narrow spectrum tetracycline-class antibiotic being developed for acne treatment is sarecycline. Along with exhibiting activity against important skin/soft tissue pathogens, sarecycline also has targeted antibacterial activity against clinical isolates of *Cutibacterium acnes*. In the current study, sarecycline was found to be 16 to 32-fold less active than broad-spectrum tetracyclines such as minocycline and doxycycline against aerobic gram-negative bacilli associated with the normal human intestinal microbiome. Sarecycline has a low propensity for resistance development in *C. acnes* strains.

COMMENT

Doxycycline is presently preferred as the first-line oral tetracycline for acne therapy as other systemic therapy methods (tetracycline and nontetracycline) such as minocycline, cotrimoxazole, quinolones, clindamycin, macrolides, and trimethoprim are associated with important side impacts and the risk of developing resistance. *C. acnes* produce proteins/enzymes that play a role in inflammation (e.g. lipase) which would also be downregulated as a consequence of inhibition of protein synthesis and accounts for the anti-inflammatory properties observed with sarecycline. Since minocycline and doxycycline display a wide range of antimicrobial activity beyond their targeted pathogens, their extensive use is connected with off-target antibacterial impacts on the human microbiome (i.e. intestinal flora) that may clinically manifest as diarrhea, fungal overgrowth (intestine and vagina) and vaginal candidiasis, particularly in patients undergoing acne treatment. This is also associated with antibiotic resistance. Sarecycline is a novel oral aminomethylcycline with a unique and stable modification at position C7 – 7-{[methoxy(methyl)amino]methyl}. The present research aimed to determine the spectrum of sarecycline and comparator tetracycline in vitro activity against both aerobic and anaerobic bacteria, including *C. acnes* and in vitro evaluation of the effectiveness, mode of action and potential for growth of resistance. Few studies evaluated the efficacy and safety of once-daily sarecycline 1.5 mg/kg for 12 weeks in patients with moderate-to-severe facial acne vulgaris. Sarecycline retains antibacterial activity against *C. acnes* and important skin pathogens such as Staphylococci, but reduced activity against aerobic enteric gram-negative bacteria as well as representative anaerobes that comprise the normal intestinal flora. The distinctive narrow spectrum of antibacterial activity of sarecyline may lead in decreased intestinal (and possibly vaginal) flora dysbiosis, resulting in decreased overgrowth of resistant bacteria and yeast infections, as well as decreased negative gastrointestinal impacts such as diarrhea. In contrast, other tetracycline-class antibiotics may be associated with gastrointestinal tract side effects, phototoxicity (typically seen with doxycycline), candidiasis, or vestibular side effects (observed with minocycline), whereas sarecycline had low rates of such side effects.

Sarecycline is the first antibiotic derived from narrow-spectrum tetracycline that may decrease the potential for gastrointestinal dysbiosis, adverse effects, and resistance growth issues during treatment.

Key Messages

- Sarecycline is a novel oral aminomethylcycline with a unique and stable modification at position C7 – 7-{[methoxy(methyl)amino]methyl}
- Sarecycline retains antibacterial activity against C. acnes and important skin pathogens such as Staphylococci, but reduced activity against aerobic enteric gram-negative bacteria as well as representative anaerobes that comprise the normal intestinal flora
- Sarecycline is the first narrow-spectrum tetracycline-derived antibiotic that may reduce the potential for gastrointestinal dysbiosis, adverse effects, and concerns regarding resistance development during therapy.

ARTICLE 99

Daily Intake of Soft Drinks and Moderate-to-severe Acne Vulgaris in Chinese Adolescents

Huang X, Zhang J, Li J, et al. Daily intake of soft drinks and moderate-to-severe acne vulgaris in Chinese adolescents. *J Pediatr.* 2019;204:256-62.

Abstract

This study investigated the association of soft drink consumption and the intake of sugar from soft drinks with the prevalence of acne in adolescents. This was a university-based epidemiologic investigation that included 8,226 students. Daily soft drink consumption with sugar intake exceeding 100 g/day significantly increased the risk of moderate-to-severe acne in adolescents.

COMMENT

High-glycemic diets may promote acne vulgaris growth or exacerbation. This study explores the association of soft drink consumption with acne in adolescents. Students from throughout the nation underwent a questionnaire survey after their enrollment in a university in Changsha, China. The daily sugar intake (grams) from soft drinks was calculated as follows: (frequency of carbonated soda consumption per week/7) × sugar content per serving + (frequency of sweetened tea drink consumption per week/7) × sugar content per serving + (frequency of fruit-flavored drink consumption per week/7) × sugar content per serving. Acne was not significantly associated with BMI, but there was a dose-response relationship with intake of sugar from any soft drinks and BMI. This study demonstrated that a high daily intake of sugar from soft drinks (≥100 g/day) was significantly associated with a 3-fold increase in the risk of moderate-to-severe acne.

There have been randomized trials confirming that a reduction in glycemic load improved the clinical symptoms of acne. Some studies have shown that nutritional patterns such as Mediterranean diet or ketogenic diet, associated by elevated fruit and vegetable intake or reduced carbohydrates and increased protein percentage, can ease acne. A high-glycemic diet can result in postprandial hyperinsulinemia and increased serum levels of free insulin like growth factor-1 (IGF-1), thus activating mammalian target of rapamycin complex 1 (mTORC1), which is nutrient sensitive. Sugar soft drinks mediate sebum synthesis and manufacturing by raising the amount of insulin and IGF-1 and activating mTORC1, and in turn foster overgrowth of *P. acnes* and create noticeable sebofollicular inflammatory acne vulgaris. There is no consensus on the relationship between BMI and acne, possibly because of errors in the measurement of sugar intake. In future studies, levels of blood glucose, insulin, IGF-1, androgen, and testosterone should be determined to better understand whether BMI mediates the effect of sugars on acne. This study also revealed that intake of fruit flavored drinks had significant protective effect against acne due to vitamin C (ascorbic acid), an essential nutrient involved in the repair of tissue and the enzymatic production of certain neurotransmitters. This study's power is that it had a comparatively large sample size and the sample had adequate geographic variation. Less frequent soft drink consumption is recommended for adolescents to prevent acne.

Key Messages

- A high-glycemic diet can result in postprandial hyperinsulinemia and increased serum levels of free insulin like growth factor-1 (IGF-1), activating mTORC1, which mediate sebum synthesis and production and in turn promote the overgrowth of *P. acnes* and develop the visible sebofollicular inflammasomopathy acne vulgaris
- Less frequent soft drink consumption is recommended for adolescents to prevent acne.

ARTICLE 100

New Concepts, Concerns, and Creations in Acne

Marson JW, Baldwin HE. New concepts, concerns, and creations in acne.
Dermatol Clin. 2019;37(1):1-9.

Abstract

In this article authors, have discussed new concepts in management of acne. Role of baseline creatinine kinase in athletes before starting oral isotretinoin therapy is discussed. Gamma-glutamyltransferase is more specific for hepatic injury due to isotretinoin. The role of light-based therapy as a single modality for acne is yet to be established. Authors have also discussed the role of microbiomes and probiotics in acne.

COMMENT

Literature on acne is replete with new concepts regarding pathophysiology and therapeutic approaches. The authors recommend baseline creatine kinase (CK) evaluation in all individuals prior to initiation of oral isotretinoin (OI) therapy. Regular monitoring of serum CK is recommended in male athletes. Patients with serum CK levels that approach or exceed five times the normal laboratory values should either stop or decrease physical activity or OI dosage. Elevated AST/ALT may originate from muscle and not liver tissue, GGT may be more specific for liver dysfunction during OI therapy.

Laser/light-based therapies (LBTs) like aminolevulinic acid photodynamic therapy (ALA-PDT) use energy to excite endogenous (porphyrins) or exogenous photosensitive adjuncts and create radical oxygen species targeted either at *Propionibacterium acnes* or the sebaceous gland, reducing inflammation and sebum production. Many of the present research have been underpowered and have not been long enough. More stringently designed studies are needed to determine the role of LBT as an adjunct or even monotherapy.

Evidence suggests there is inherent epidermal barrier dysfunction in acne-prone skin, creating an inhospitable environment for commensal species. This imbalance generates permissible circumstances for the infection and inflammation of pathological strains such as *Propionibacterium acnes*. Studies suggest that probiotics (commensal species) and prebiotics which are nonliving substances that promote beneficial bacteria, may have therapeutic potential against acne by mending the epidermal barrier. It was discovered that people with acne had a decrease in inflammatory lesions and sebum content and reduced triacylglycerol content after 12 weeks of consuming fermented milk with 200 mg of lactoferrin than people with acne who only consumed fermented milk. Genetic factors likely predetermine the inflammatory response and ultimately the wound healing process resulting from the trauma of the acne lesion. Atrophic acne scars, are actually active and dynamic lesions. Acne relapse has been correlated with scar development after original successful therapy, enhanced body mass index (BMI), male gender, and a favorable family history of severe acne, with delay in treatment being the most consistent and substantial risk factor. Fillers, laser, chemical and mechanical resurfacing techniques, microneedling, and surgical interventions (subcision and excisional techniques) have been shown to improve, but not normalize, the appearance of scars. Topical retinoids in photographed skin have been shown to enhance fine lines and wrinkles, probably due to their capacity to boost procollagen fibroblast development. New therapies that target the inflammatory cascade and sebum suppression, oral antibiotics with a narrow spectrum of activity, topical antibacterials with less risk of resistance and without systemic absorption, and probiotics are all in various stages of clinical development. Topical minocycline, topical nitric oxide gels are all in the pipeline. Sarecycline is an antibiotic tetracycline-class with a narrow spectrum of activity targeting *P. acnes* and *Staphylococcus aureus* and more restricted activity against gastrointestinal gram-negative bacteria than minocycline and doxycycline. Trifarotene is the first fourth-generation retinoid to be studied for acne vulgaris which is a highly selective retinoic acid receptor-gamma (RAR-ϒ) agonist, which could potentially increase efficacy and/or decrease irritation compared with the less selective agents. Cortexalone 17α-propionate 1% cream with certain anti-inflammatory characteristics is a topical peripherally selective steroidal antiandrogen. It has been shown to easily penetrate human skin, where it is metabolized into cortexolone, which lacks androgenic effects.

Key Messages

- Creatine kinase should be monitored in athletic males on isotretinoin
- Gamma-glutamyltransferase is superior to other liver transaminases when following hepatic function of isotretinoin
- Acne scarring is partly a result of delayed and inadequate treatment
- The acne pipeline is rich with new chemical entities and combinations
- Laser and light therapies for acne, while effective, need additional evidence-based data to support their use as a first-line therapy.

ARTICLE 101

The Anti-inflammatory Activities of *Propionibacterium acnes* CAMP Factor-targeted Acne Vaccines

Wang Y, Hata TR, Tong YL, et al. The Anti-Inflammatory Activities of *Propionibacterium acnes* CAMP Factor-targeted Acne Vaccines.
J Invest Dermatol. 2018;138(11):2355-64.

Abstract
Secretory Christie-Atkins-Munch-Petersen (CAMP) factor of *Propionibacterium acnes* is upregulated in anaerobic cultures and plays an essential role in the cytotoxicity of *P. acnes*. Vaccination of mice with CAMP factor considerably reduced the growth of *P. acnes* and production of MIP-2, a murine counterpart of human IL-8. The authors found that *P. acnes* CAMP factor and two proinflammatory cytokines (IL-8 and IL-1β) were expressed at higher levels in acne lesions than those in nonlesional skin.

COMMENT

Current treatments for acne target the *P. acnes* organism, which has been implicated in the genesis of inflammation in acne. In this study, the authors used a vaccination approach to test whether *P. acnes* Christie-Atkins-Munch-Petersen (CAMP) factor, a secretory virulence factor, is a main source of inflammation in acne vulgaris. *Propionibacterium acnes* CAMP factor is able to bind to immunoglobulin G and M classes and acts as a pore-forming toxin. Here they studied the use of a particular secretory virulence factor as a vaccine because it has been stated that there is less selective pressure for resistant bacteria to develop particular inhibition of secretory virulence factors. Upregulation of *P. acnes* CAMP factor occurs under anaerobic conditions. Experimental results also showed the requirement of CAMP factor for *P. acnes*-induced inflammation. Vaccination with *P. acnes* CAMP factor with aluminum as adjuvant elicited protective immunity against *P. acnes*. The CAMP factor was detected in hair follicles and sebaceous glands in nonlesional skin whereas it was distributed everywhere in an acne lesion.

The CAMP factor acts as a pore forming toxin that may induce cytolysis and cytokine secretion via activation of the inflammasome. Also, it has been shown that CAMP factor 2, but not 4, is the major active co-hemolytic factor of *P. acnes*. No conclusive proof shows the correlation between CAMP factor expression and acne severity and the role of CAMP factor in acne vulgaris pathogenesis. *Propionibacterium acnes* bacteria play a key role in the development of inflammatory lesions via induction of secretion of IL-6 and IL-8 by follicular keratinocytes, IL-1β, tumor necrosis factor-α, IL-8, and IL-12 by monocytic cells in a toll-like receptor 2-dependent manner. *Propionibacterium acnes* bacteria triggered mixed Th17/Th1 reactions by causing concurrent secretion from particular CD4 T cells of IL-17A and IFN-rates. If the humanized mAb to CAMP factor can be developed, the injection of the mAb to CAMP factor directly into acne lesions potentially can replace triamcinolone acetonide for intralesional therapy against acne vulgaris.

Key Messages

- Christie-Atkins-Munch-Petersen (CAMP) factor, a secretory virulence factor, is a main source of inflammation in acne vulgaris
- CAMP factor acts as a pore forming toxin that may induce cytolysis and cytokine secretion via activation of the inflammasome
- If the humanized mAb to CAMP factor can be developed, the injection of the mAb to CAMP factor directly into acne lesions potentially can be an intralesional therapy against acne vulgaris.

ARTICLE 102

Skin Ecology during Sebaceous Drought—How Skin Microbes Respond to Isotretinoin

McCoy WH 4th, Otchere E, Rosa BA, et al. Skin ecology during sebaceous drought—how skin microbes respond to isotretinoin.
J Invest Dermatol. 2019;139(3):732-5.

Abstract

Acne is commonly treated either with isotretinoin or antibiotics. The authors hypothesized that successful acne treatment with isotretinoin would shift an "acne microbiome" to resemble that found in normal skin. A pilot observational, prospective study comparing isotretinoin-treated acne subjects versus two untreated control groups (normal skin, acne) was performed. Cutibacterium *acnes* globally declined throughout treatment.

COMMENT

Acne antibiotics target *Cutibacterium* (formerly *Propionibacterium*) *acnes* (*C. acnes*). This bacterium is associated with acne and can cause opportunistic infections. Prolonged antibiotics can cause significant collateral damage like dysbiosis and antibiotic resistance. Isotretinoin, a non-antimicrobial, systemic retinoid improves acne in most patients by decreasing sebum and *C. acnes* levels. The authors performed a pilot observational, prospective study comparing isotretinoin-treated acne subjects versus two untreated control groups (normal skin, acne). Acne severity (Global Evaluation Acne score), skin sampling, control samples, targeted metagenomic next-generation sequencing (16S rRNA gene V1eV2 hypervariable region), and genomic analyses were performed. All available skin swabs (88) from 17 isotretinoin-treated subjects and 8 untreated control individuals (4 normal skin, 4 acne) underwent initial processing.

Cutibacterium acnes globally declined throughout treatment. *Staphylococcus* species increased initially but then decreased before treatment completion. The authors suggest that isotretinoin creates a *Propionibacterium* "population bottleneck" that selects for "healthy" *Propionibacterium* communities and other sebaceous skin taxa that persist after treatment, resulting in long-term acne remission. This work should inspire future studies leading to the development of "prebiotic fertilizers," strain-selective "weed killers," and/or probiotic *Propionibacterium* strains that optimize pilosebaceous unit PSU ecosystems while avoiding antibiotic "collateral damage."

Key Messages
- Prolonged antibiotics to treat acne can cause significant collateral damage like dysbiosis and antibiotic resistance
- Isotretinoin, a non-antimicrobial, systemic retinoid improves acne in most patients by decreasing sebum and C. acnes levels.

ARTICLE 103

Propionibacterium acnes-derived Extracellular Vesicles Promote Acne-like Phenotypes in Human Epidermis

Choi EJ, Lee HG, Bae IH, et al. *Propionibacterium acnes*-derived extracellular vesicles promote acne-like phenotypes in human epidermis.
J Invest Dermatol. 2018;138(6):1371-9.

Abstract

Propionibacterium acnes-derived extracellular vesicles (PEVs) can induce acne-like phenotypes in human epidermal keratinocytes. Inflammatory cytokines IL-8 and GM-CSF are induced by them, and they also dysregulate epidermal differentiation by increasing proliferating keratinocytes and decreasing epidermal keratin 10 and desmocollin 1 levels. The authors verified that PEVs were internalized via clathrin-dependent endocytosis into keratinocytes and cellular responses occurred via TLR2-dependent signal cascades. Inhibiting the release of EVs from *P. acnes* or targeting PEV-mediated signaling pathways could represent an alternative method for alleviating acne occurrence and phenotypes.

COMMENT

It is found that substantial heritable genetic factors contribute to acne susceptibility and determine its occurrence. Various factors such as ethnicity, hormones, diet, sunlight, smoking, stress, obesity, and infection are also thought to be related to acne pathogenesis. Although *P. acnes* is predicted to play roles in acne pathogenesis, the exact mechanism of action at the molecular level has not been clarified. Most of these bacteria release extracellular vesicles (EVs) known as outer membrane vesicles and membrane vesicles which are lipid bilayer-enclosed spherical vesicles approximately 30–1,000 nm in diameter. Bacterial EVs are known to mediate pathophysiological functions in bacteria–bacteria and bacteria–host interactions by delivering toxins, inducing cellular inflammation, and evoking host cell death.

The authors found that *Propionibacterium acnes*-derived extracellular vesicles (PEVs) induce acne-like phenotypes such as increased secretion of inflammatory cytokines and dysregulated epidermal differentiation via TLR2-mediated signaling pathways. They demonstrated that entry of PEVs into keratinocytes is mediated by clathrin-dependent endocytosis and that the internal cargo of PEVs can be delivered into host cells. PEVs upregulate the expression of proinflammatory cytokines in the human epidermis, independently of *P. acnes*, and thus participate in inflammatory reactions by stimulating keratinocytes in acne lesions. PEVs affect the expression of epidermal markers related to proliferation and differentiation and result in epidermal deformation including hyperkeratinization. PEVs induce fast and intense inflammatory cytokine production and more efficiently reduce epidermal differentiation markers than *P. acnes* extracts. TLR2 is a major receptor for PEVs in human keratinocytes and mediates PEV-induced cellular responses. PEVs significantly increase the secretion of cytokines such as IL-8, GM-CSF, CXCL1, and CXCL5, promoting the infiltration of neutrophils. PEVs stimulate both keratinocytes and myeloid cells, and cells associated with the immune system may be more susceptible than epidermal keratinocytes to PEV stimulation. In summary, this study suggests that lipid bilayer-enclosed and nanosized PEVs efficiently induce not only inflammatory responses but also epidermal deformation, i.e. acne-like phenotypes. Therefore, the targeting of PEV-mediated pathogenesis using neutralizing antibodies against PEV-induced cytokines and TLR2 or the inhibition of the release of EVs from *P. acnes* could be alternative methods for alleviating acne occurrence and phenotypes.

Key Messages

- *P. acnes-derived EVs (PEVs) induce acne-like phenotypes such as increased secretion of inflammatory cytokines and dysregulated epidermal differentiation via TLR2-mediated signaling pathways*
- *Targeting of PEV-mediated pathogenesis using neutralizing antibodies against PEV-induced cytokines and TLR2 or the inhibition of the release of EVs from P. acnes could be alternative methods for alleviating acne occurrence.*

ARTICLE 104

Patients with Acne Vulgaris have a Distinct Gut Microbiota in Comparison with Healthy Controls

Deng Y, Wang H, Zhou J, et al. Patients with acne vulgaris have a distinct gut microbiota in comparison with healthy controls.
Acta Derm Venereol. 2018;98(7-8):783-90.

Abstract

Acne vulgaris has been considered to have a gastrointestinal mechanism; however, not much is known about gut microbiota dysfunction in this condition. The present study was a cross-sectional study to investigate whether the gut microbiota is altered in acne. Fecal bacterial diversity was analyzed in patients with acne and healthy controls. Significant differences were found in microbial diversity between patients with acne and controls. However, further larger studies can be done to assess its role in the pathogenesis of acne.

COMMENT

Acne vulgaris is a chronic inflammatory disease of the pilosebaceous units. There is a significant role of *P. acnes* in the inflammation. The role of western diet has been studied in the pathogenesis of acne. Altered gut microbiota has been considered to have a role in the pathogenesis of acne. However, there is no direct evidence.

A total of 43 patients with acne vulgaris and 43 age-and sex-matched controls were recruited for the study. All the participants were questioned about their dietary habits in the last 6 months. Fresh stool samples were collected from all the participants in a sterile container. The 16S rDNA gene amplification and sequencing were done from the samples.

This study shows that the composition of gut microbiota in patients with acne differs significantly from that in healthy controls. There was a reduced diversity of gut microbiota in patients with acne which is seen in other inflammatory skin diseases like Behcet's and psoriasis. At the phylum level, the abundance of *Firmicutes* was lower in the patient group, but that of *Bacteroidiain* was higher. The most significantly depleted taxa in acne were *Clostridia, Clostridiales, Lachnospiraceae* and *Ruminococcaceae* genera, which are potentially beneficial. This altered microbiota could lead to change in the intestinal epithelial barrier and lead to altered immune response releasing inflammatory cytokines. In conclusion, patients with acne vulgaris have gut microbial dysbiosis; further study is needed to understand its role in the pathogenesis of acne.

Key Messages
- *There is a difference in gut microbiota between acne patients and healthy controls*
- *Reduced diversity of gut microbiota is seen in patients with acne*
- *Role of western diet in development of acne is validated in this study.*

ARTICLE 105

Inhibitory Effects of *Euphorbia supina* on *Propionibacterium acnes*-induced Skin Inflammation In Vitro and In Vivo

Lim HJ, Jeon YD, Kang SH, et al. Inhibitory effects of *Euphorbia supina* on *Propionibacterium acnes*-induced skin inflammation in vitro and in vivo.
BMC Complement Altern Med. 2018;18(1):263.

Abstract

The study was done to determine the antibacterial and anti-inflammatory activities of *Euphorbia supina* (ES) against *P. acnes*, the etiologic agent of skin inflammation. The tests were conducted both in vitro and in vivo. Various methods were used to look for the antibacterial and anti-inflammatory activity of ES. Proinflammatory cytokines were assessed. The study demonstrates the antibacterial and anti-inflammatory activities of ES extract against *P. acnes*. The ES extract might be used to treat inflammatory skin disease.

COMMENT

Acne is an inflammatory disorder of the pilosebaceous unit. *Propionibacterium acnes* plays a major role in the inflammatory response in acne by stimulating toll-like receptor 2. Suppressing *P. acnes* induced inflammation is one of the major targets for treating acne vulgaris.

Euphorbia supina (ES) plant has been used in herbal medications for its antioxidant, anti-arthritic, detoxification, diuretic and hemostatic effects on various cell types. The active substances include tannins, terpenoids and polyphenols.

This study was done to detect the antibacterial and anti-inflammatory effects of ES in the in vitro model and also in the living *P. acnes* induced acne skin disease model. This was tested using disc diffusion and broth dilution method. MTT assay was done to evaluate the cytotoxicity of ES at different doses. The proinflammatory cytokines and mRNA levels were measured by ELISA and real-time PCR. The chemical composition of ES was analyzed by liquid chromatography-mass spectrometry (LC-MS).

A strong antibacterial activity against *P. acnes* and inhibitory activity on lipase was detected in ES. However, it did not have significant cytotoxicity on THP-1 cells. ES inhibited the expression levels of pro-inflammatory cytokines and the MAPK signaling pathway. Protocatechuic acid, gallic acid, quercetin, and kaempferol were detected in ES. It also reduced the inflammation and ear thickness in the mouse model injected with *P. acnes* extract to the ear.

This study demonstrates the antibacterial and anti-inflammatory activities of ES extract against *P. acnes*. The ES extract might be used to treat anti-inflammatory skin disease.

Key Messages
- The ES extract has a strong antibacterial activity against P. acnes
- The ES extract suppressed proinflammatory cytokines and MAPK signaling pathway
- The ES extract inhibited inflammation in a mice model of acnes induced by intradermal injection of P. acnes
- The ES extract might be used in the treatment of inflammatory skin disease.

ARTICLE 106

Isolation and Identification of the Follicular Microbiome: Implications for Acne Research

Hall JB, Cong Z, Imamura-Kawasawa Y, et al. Isolation and identification of the follicular microbiome: Implications for acne research.
J Invest Dermatol. 2018;138(9):2033-40.

Abstract

The role of *P. acnes* in skin homeostasis and acne pathogenesis is being extensively studied. Various methods for sampling and identifying the skin's microbiome exist. The present study aims to compare the microbial diversity of samples obtained from the cheeks of 20 volunteers, collected by surface swab, pore strips, and cyanoacrylate glue follicular biopsy. The 16S rRNA sequencing (V1-V3) and whole-genome metagenomic sequencing (WGS) were used to detect the microbial flora. WGS detected more species diversity including viruses. However, the overall diversity did not differ between sampling methods. The identification of *P. acnes* bacteria, ribotypes, and bacteriophages were equal by all sampling methods indicating that all may be equally useful for acne-related research studies.

COMMENT

The role of skin microbiome in the healthy and disease states is an area of active research. Acne vulgaris is a disease of the pilosebaceous unit, and the microbiome samples should be collected from within the follicle. Earlier studies have used the commercially available pore strips to sample the follicular niche from the nose of acne patients. However, there are not many studies comparing the various sampling methods and sequencing techniques in the same group of patients. The sampling and the sequencing method can cause variation in the detection and identification of the microbiome.

This is a split face study where the samples were taken using three different methods—cotton swabs, commercially available pore strips and cyanoacrylate glue follicular biopsies and multiple sequencing methods and whole genome sequencing. Twenty seven volunteers in the age group of 12–40 years with normal to mild facial acne were recruited for the study. Two cohorts were made A and B. Pore stripping on the right cheek and glue follicular biopsy on the left cheek was used in cohort A whereas cotton swab on right cheek and glue follicular biopsy on the left cheek was used in cohort B.

Depth of follicular sampling—complete follicles were isolated by glue method whereas the casts isolated by pore strips were incomplete and broken. Hence better follicular depth was obtained using glue method. Also, some patients preferred the glue method as there was less drying.

All samples were sequenced using 16S V1 to V3 and whole gene sequencing. There was no difference in the diversity in the follicle sampling method regardless of the sequencing method used. *Propionibacterium acnes* was the most abundant species detected. However, the viral composition of the skin's surface is unique compared to the follicle, suggesting distinct viral niches within the skin. Both follicular sampling methods identified the follicular microbiome was equally effective for each method.

> **Key Messages**
> - The overall diversity of organisms does not differ between sampling methods
> - Sequencing methods influence the detection microbial profiles
> - WGS capture more species diversity including viruses compared to 16S rRNA sequencing.

ARTICLE 107

Expression of Inflammatory and Fibrogenetic Markers in Acne Hypertrophic Scar Formation: Focusing on Role of TGF-β and IGF-1R

Yang JH, Yoon JY, Moon J, et al. Expression of inflammatory and fibrogenetic markers in acne hypertrophic scar formation: focusing on role of TGF-β and IGF-1R.
Arch Dermatol Res. 2018;310(8):665-73.

Abstract

Acne vulgaris is a common skin disease which can heal with scars. Acne scars can cause significant cosmetic and psychological problems, leading to poor quality of life. The scars can be atrophic or hypertrophic. This study was done to investigate the role of fibrogenetic and inflammatory markers in the pathogenesis of hypertrophic scars. Immunohistochemistry staining and quantitative PCR were performed for fibrogenetic and inflammatory markers in the skin biopsy samples taken from the hypertrophic scars and normal skin. Vimentin and α-SMA were increased in both mature and immature hypertrophic scars. Also, the production of TGF-β3 protein and its transcription was also significantly elevated. Expression levels of SMAD2 and SMAD4 were increased. Elevation of these factors may give clues for acne hypertrophic scar formation.

COMMENT

Acne is one of the most common skin conditions in adolescents and young adults. Moderate-to-severe acne can cause scarring leading to significant cosmetic and psychological morbidity. The scars can be atrophic or hypertrophic. There have been various studies on the treatment of acne scars, however not many studies regarding understanding the pathogenesis of acne scars. The present study was done to detect the underlying pathogenesis of hypertrophic acne scars by checking the roles of fibrogenic and inflammatory markers using immunohistochemistry and quantitative PCR.

A total of 12 patients with acne scar were recruited for the study. Both mature and immature hypertrophic acne scars were considered for the study. Punches measuring 3 mm and 4 mm were used to take skin biopsy from the area of hypertrophic acne scar on the face and back respectively and also from the normal skin as control group.

Immunohistochemistry was performed for the following molecules: TGF-β1, TGF-β3, IGF-1R, insulin-degrading enzyme (IDE), CD45RA, CD45RO, CD26, CD44, CK-14, α-SMA, vimentin, IL-1α, IL-1β, IL-4, IL-10, TNF-α, MMP-3, SMAD2, SMAD4 and MMP-1. IQ solution program was used to measure the intensity of the immunohistochemistry staining. Also quantitative PCR was done with primer sequences of TGF-β1, TGF-β3, IL-1α, IL-1β, IL-10, TNF-α, MMP-1 and MMP-3. The results showed higher immunoreactivity to vimentin and alpha smooth muscle actin compared to normal skin. Also, TGF-β3 expression was higher in mature hypertrophic scars. SMAD2 and SMAD4 were increased in the scars of the face only and not over the back. CD45RO expression was increased in mature hypertrophic scar. The quantitative PCR results were consistent with findings of immunohistochemistry staining.

Immature hypertrophic scars showed increased expression of IGF-1R and IDE in the dermis. SMAD2 and SMAD4 were also increased. In addition, apoptosis was increased in immature hypertrophic scars compared to adjacent normal skin. Abnormal reaction in wound healing can lead to excessive collagen deposition and hence hypertrophic scarring. In the present study, TGF-β3 was increased compared to TGF-β1. The profibrotic factors might be more active than the antifibrotic pathway causing excessive fibrosis of skin. Downstream signaling molecules of TGF-β can be targeted as new therapeutic option to prevent acne scars. Increase in CD45RO, TNF-α and IL–4 shows that inflammation is in progress in mature hypertrophic scars and exaggerated inflammation might increase the profibrotic cytokines. Increased expression of vimentin and smooth muscle actin and reduced MMP indicate the proliferation of fibroblasts and myofibroblasts.

Key Messages

- TGF-β3 is elevated in hypertrophic acne scars compared to TGF-β1 in other hypertrophic scars
- Newer therapeutic options targeting the underlying pathomechanisms can be developed to prevent and treat hypertrophic acne scars.

ARTICLE 108

Decrease in Diversity of *Propionibacterium acnes* Phylotypes in Patients with Severe Acne on the Back

Dagnelie MA, Corvec S, Saint-Jean M, et al. Decrease in diversity of *Propionibacterium acnes* phylotypes in patients with severe acne on the back.
Acta Derm Venereol. 2018;98(1-2):262-7.

Abstract

Propionibacterium acnes, one of the main causative factors in acne is subdivided into six phylotypes: IA1, IA2, IB, IC, II and III. This study detected *P. acnes* subgroups on the face and back of patients with severe acne and in healthy controls. *Propionibacterium acnes* phylotypes were identical on the face and back in 71.4% of patients with severe acne, whereas 45.5% of healthy controls had such distribution. There was a high predominance of IA1 (84.4%), especially on the back (95.6%) in patients with acne. Also, the single-locus sequence typing (SLST) method revealed A1 to be the predominant type on the back of patients with acne, compared with a wide diversity in the healthy group. Hence, this study reports that severity of acne on the back is associated with loss of diversity of *P. acnes* phylotype, with a major predominance of phylotype IA1. This change might be an inducing factor in the activation of *P. acnes*, which could trigger inflammation.

COMMENT

Acne is one of the most common skin diseases affecting 85% of the population. *Propionibacterium acnes* which is an anaerobic gram-positive bacterium, plays an important role in pathogenesis of acne. It is more specifically located in the pilosebaceous follicle. It activates inflammation through toll-like receptor 2 and stimulates secretion of various inflammatory cytokines. *Propionibacterium acnes* is divided into six phylotypes: IA1, IA2, IB, IC, II and III. The objective of this study was to detect and compare different *P. acnes* phylotypes, clonal complexes, and single locus sequence types on the face and back of patients with severe acne over the back and in healthy controls.

Patients with severe acne and healthy controls were recruited for the study after considering the inclusion and exclusion criteria. Acne scoring was done using Groupe Expert Acne scale. Swabs were taken from the face and back of all the study participants. Anaerobic culture was done for 7-10 days. DNA extraction was done from all isolates and six main phylotypes were determined. Multilocus sequence typing (MLST) and single-locus sequence typing (SLST) was done to look for the clonal complexes. A total of 24 patients and 12 healthy volunteers participated in the study. Culture was positive in all the cases. Other than *P. acnes*, different species like *P. avidum*, *P. granulosum* and

P. namnetense were also isolated. There was no significant difference in bacterial diversity in the face samples from acne patients and healthy subjects.

Healthy subjects showed a large diversity in phenotypes. The main types were phylotype IA1 and II. In acne patients, phylotype IA1 was the main type (84.4%) both over the face and back.

The SLST type A1 was the predominant type in the acne group. Few newer SLST types were also identified which was not described earlier like K16 (phylotype II) and L7 (phylotype III) in healthy groups; A27, A289 (phylotype IA1), F11 (phylotype IA2), K17 (phylotype II).

The study shows that there is a loss of diversity of *P. acnes* phylotypes in acne patients with a higher predominance of phylotype IA1. Also, SLST type A1 was the predominant type found in nodular acne over the back. Probably this loss of diversity could activate the innate immunity and trigger the inflammation in acne.

Key Messages
- There are six major phylotypes of Propionibacterium acnes
- Severity of back acne may be associated with loss of diversity in P. acnes phylotypes
- Altered balance of P. acnes phylotypes might be an inducing factor in inflammation.

ARTICLE 109

Short Lipopeptides Specifically Inhibit the Growth of *Propionibacterium acnes* with Antibacterial and Anti-inflammatory Dual Action

Yang G, Wang J, Lu S, et al. Short lipopeptides specifically inhibit the growth of *Propionibacterium acnes* with antibacterial and anti-inflammatory dual action.
Br J Pharmacol. 2019;176(11):1603-8.

Abstract

Propionibacterium acnes (*P. acnes*), a gram-positive bacterium is an important factor in the pathogenesis of acne vulgaris. Fatty acids play an important role in the life habitat of *P. acnes*. The present study aims to look for short lipopeptides with potent antimicrobial action against *P. acnes*. Minimal inhibitory concentration (MIC) was used to determine antimicrobial activity of various peptides. RAW264.7 cells stimulated with LPS and *P. acnes* were used to measure the anti-inflammatory activity. Mice ears injected with *P. acnes* were used to assess the antimicrobial and anti-inflammatory effects of tested peptides in vivo.

> C16-KWKW was the most potent candidate among the various lipopeptides with a MIC of 2 μg/mL. The mode of action of C16-KWKW was by impairing membrane permeability and causing leakage of inner contents of bacterial cells. Also, it inhibited the expression of pro-inflammatory cytokines, such as IL-1β, TNF-α, and iNOS stimulated by both LPS and *P. acnes*, thus showing potential anti-inflammatory activity. Hence, the lipopeptide C16-KWKW having both anti-*P. acnes* and anti-inflammatory action in vitro and in vivo can have a potential role in the treatment of acne vulgaris.

COMMENT

Acne vulgaris is a chronic skin disorder having an emotional and psychological impact. *Propionibacterium acnes* has a key role in the pathogenesis of acne and associated inflammation. *Propionibacterium acnes* is known to induce release of proinflammatory cytokines like IL-1β, IL-8 and TNF-α which plays a major role in the acne pathogenesis.

Various therapeutic options are there which acts on different stages of acne development. Use of antimicrobial peptides is a newer approach due to its rapid action and also reduced chances of resistance. This study investigates the development of potent anti-*P. acnes* peptides with antimicrobial and anti-inflammatory effect.

An anti-*P. acnes* peptide library was developed and modified by conjugating a peptide KWKW with various lengths of fatty acids. Among the different peptides, C16-KWKW showed a potent and specific anti-*P. acnes* activity which was checked by employing the MIC. The activity was more specific against *P. acnes* which was confirmed by quantitative real-time PCR. This peptide also showed a faster killing kinetics compared to clindamycin. The evaluation of cytotoxicity showed no significant toxicity. It also had an effect on the expression of proinflammatory cytokines secreted by LPS and *P. acnes*.

The antimicrobial action of this peptide was shown to be via interfering with bacterial membrane of *P. acnes*. This damages the bacterial cell membrane and causes the leakage of inner components. This was assessed using transmission electron microscopy, nucleic acid leakage measurement, and PI uptake assay.

Key Messages

- C16-KWKW, a lipopeptide exhibiting potent anti-*P. acnes* and anti-inflammatory activities both in vitro and in vivo
- It is more active against *P. acnes* than other bacteria, and shows faster killing kinetics. Even the toxicity level is low. Hence, this short lipopeptide can be a promising therapeutic option in acne vulgaris.

ARTICLE 110

Plasma Exeresis for Active Acne Vulgaris: Clinical and In Vivo Microscopic Documentation of Treatment Efficacy by Means of Reflectance Confocal Microscopy

Rossi E, Mandel VD, Paganelli A, et al. Plasma exeresis for active acne vulgaris: Clinical and in vivo microscopic documentation of treatment efficacy by means of reflectance confocal microscopy.
Skin Res Technol. 2018;24(3):522-4.

Abstract

Acne is a chronic disorder of pilosebaceous glands which sometimes requires long-term therapy. The most common cause for failure of therapy is nonadherence to treatment. The authors have studied the effects of plasma exeresis for active acne and reported complete clearance of the lesions in 6 months. This could be a useful therapy for patients who are not compliant with topical and systemic therapy.

COMMENT

The most common cause for treatment failure in acne is noncompliance with therapy. Oral antibiotics and oral isotretinoin is prescribed for 2-4 months to control the initial flare of acne. As acne is a chronic disorder, sometimes patients will need to take therapy for long time for maintenance of remission. Physical modalities like laser, photodynamic therapy are better alternative for patients who do not follow or cannot tolerate the topical therapies. In this study plasma exeresis was done for active acne, the results evaluated with confocal microscopy at the beginning of therapy and then after 6 months. Plasma exeresis was done every 2 weeks for 2 months under topical anesthesia. The treatment was followed-up with strict sun protection. Comedones were sublimated with single spot mode, pustules with single spots on periphery and papules with single spots on periphery and on central area.

There were no side effects noted at the end of the study and there was complete disappearance of lesions.

Key Message

- Plasma exeresis is a useful alternate modality of treatment for patients who do not tolerate or maintain topical therapy for acne.

ARTICLE 111

Licochalcone A Attenuates Acne Symptoms Mediated by Suppression of NLRP3 Inflammasome

Yang G, Lee HE, Yeon SH, et al. Licochalcone A attenuates acne symptoms mediated by suppression of NLRP3 inflammasome.
Phytother Res. 2018;32(12):2551-9.

Abstract

The NLRP3 inflammasome by *Propionibacterium acnes* (*P. acnes*) has an important role in the pathogenesis of acne vulgaris. *Propionibacterium acnes* secretes inflammasomes like NLRP3 which induces inflammation and aggravates development of acne lesions. This study tried to evaluate the role of Licochalcone A, a chalconoid isolated from the root of *Glycyrrhiza inflata* in inhibiting *P. acnes*-induced NLRP3 inflammasome activation. Licochalcone A blocked *P. acnes*-induced production of caspase-1 (p10) and IL-1β in primary mouse macrophages and human SZ95 sebocytes, indicating the suppression of NLRP3 inflammasome. Licochalcone A suppressed *P. acnes*-induced ASC speck formation and mitochondrial reactive oxygen species. Topical application of licochalcone A to mouse ear skin attenuated *P. acnes*-induced skin inflammation. This study has shown that licochalcone A is effective in the control of *P. acnes*-induced skin inflammation as an efficient inhibitor for NLRP3 inflammasome.

COMMENT

Acne occurs in more than 70-80% of adolescents and young adults. It can lead to scarring and hyperpigmentation causing psychological morbidity. *Propionibacterium acnes* is a well-known etiological factor for acne, however, the role of inflammasome activation by *P. acnes* is a newer concept. In the pathogenesis of acne, *P. acnes* induces the secretion of interleukin-1 beta (IL-1 beta) and NLRP3 inflammasome which have an important role in inducing inflammation and aggravation of acne lesions. One of the study reports targeting of these inflammasome could be a newer treatment option in treating acne vulgaris.

On searching for molecules which could inhibit the NLRP3 inflammosome, licochalcone A, a chalconoid isolated from the root of *Glycyrrhiza inflata*, was reported to have anti-inflammatory activity. It mainly inhibited IL-1β mediated inflammation. However, it is not clear if licochalcone A would modulate the process of IL-1β production, which is mediated by NLRP3 inflammasome.

This study tried to investigate if licochalcone A inhibits *P. acnes*-induced NLRP3 inflammasome activation and in turn if topical application of licochalcone A could be effective in treating inflammatory acne. Licochalcone A suppressed *P. acnes*-induced ASC speck formation and mitochondrial reactive oxygen species. Topical application of licochalcone A to mouse ear skin attenuated *P. acnes*-induced skin inflammation. This study has shown that licochalcone A is effective in the control of *P. acnes*-induced skin inflammation as an efficient inhibitor for NLRP3 inflammasome.

Key Messages

- Activation of the NLRP3 inflammasome by P. acnes is important in inflammatory acne
- Licochalcone A, a chalconoid isolated from the root of Glycyrrhiza inflata, was an effective inhibitor NLRP3 inflammasome activation
- The NLRP3 inflammasome could be a new target for the development of anti-acne therapy.

ARTICLE 112

Gut Microbiota Alterations in Moderate-to-severe Acne Vulgaris Patients

Yan HM, Zhao HJ, Guo DY, et al. Gut microbiota alterations in moderate to severe acne vulgaris patients.
J Dermatol. 2018;45(10):1166-71.

Abstract

Acne vulgaris is a chronic inflammatory disorder of the pilosebaceous unit. The pathogenesis is multifactorial. Few studies have indicated the role of gut microbia in the pathogenesis of acne. This study tries to detect the link between acne vulgaris and gut microbiota. Thirty-one patients of moderate to severe acne and 31 healthy controls were included in the study. Feces were collected and gut microbiota was evaluated using high-throughput sequencing. It showed a link between acne and changes in gut microbiota. *Actinobacteria* was decreased and *Proteobacteria* increased in acne patients. *Bifidobacterium, Butyricicoccus, Coprobacillus, Lactobacillus* and *Allobaculum* were all decreased. This study provides a new insight to the association between acne and gut microbiota.

COMMENT

Acne vulgaris is a chronic inflammatory disorder affecting the pilosebaceous units. It is commonly seen in adolescents and young adults. The pathogenesis of acne is multifactorial. One study from China has shown a higher prevalence of gastrointestinal symptoms in patients with acne vulgaris. Few studies have reported that gut microbiota may play a role in the pathogenesis of acne vulgaris. This study was done to check if alteration in gut microbiota had any role in pathogenesis of acne.

Thirty-one patients with moderate-to-severe acne and 31 healthy controls were recruited for the study. History of smoking and alcohol was taken from the participants.

Patients with history of inflammatory bowel disease, any other systemic disease, taking systemic corticosteroids, antibiotics, and immunosuppressive drugs were excluded from the study. Fecal samples were collected in sterile containers and stored at −20 degrees. The samples were evaluated using high-throughput sequencing to detect the bacteria DNA. Statistical analysis was done using SPSS version 20.0 to determine the statistical difference between the two groups.

At the phylum level, *Bacteroidetes*, *Firmicutes*, *Proteobacteria* and *Actinobacteria* were the main four phyla that consisted of the gut microbiota. *Proteobacteria* was higher in acne patients while *Actinobacteria* was lower.

On analyzing the genus *Bifidobacterium*, *Butyricicoccus*, *Coprobacillus*, *Lactobacillus* and *Allobaculum* were all decreased in acne patients.

Earlier studies have also shown similar results. It has been speculated that changes in the gut microbiota and reduced butyrate production can lead to dysfunction of intestinal epithelial barrier and also anti-inflammation mechanisms thus aggravating acne vulgaris. Still the exact mechanisms are not clear and needs further investigation. Also the limitations of this study include; incomplete information regarding acne subtype and other factor affecting gut microbiota like lifestyle and nutrition was not considered. Also this study was conducted in a small sample size of Chinese patients and hence difficult to extrapolate to larger groups.

Key Messages
- Gut microbiota are implicated in the pathogenesis of acne vulgaris. They are postulated to cause dysfunction of intestinal epithelial barrier and anti-inflammatory mechanisms leading to aggravation of acne
- Lifestyle and nutrition may play a role in alteration of gut microbiota which has to be considered.

ARTICLE 113

Overall and Subgroup Prevalence of Acne Vulgaris among Patients with Hidradenitis Suppurativa

Wertenteil S, Strunk A, Garg A. Overall and subgroup prevalence of acne vulgaris among patients with hidradenitis suppurativa.
J Am Acad Dermatol. 2019;80(5):1308-13.

Abstract

The burden of acne vulgaris (AV) in adults with Hidradenitis suppurativa (HS) is not known and also the evidence establishing a link between AV and HS is limited. Hence this cross-sectional study was done to estimate the prevalence of AV among adults with HS and determine the strength of this association. The study was done using electronic health record data from a population-based sample. As per this study, the prevalence of AV among adults with HS was 15.2% (7,315 of 48,085) compared with 2.9% for adults without HS. Also the prevalence was higher in patients with HS who were females, in the age group of 18–44 years, non-white, obese and having polycystic ovarian disease. HS patients had higher chances of having acne compared to patients without HS. However, the study could not assess the influence of disease severity in HS, or in acne on the strength of association.

COMMENT

Hidradenitis suppurativa (HS) is a chronic inflammatory disorder of the follicular unit presenting with painful nodules, abscesses, fistulas, sinus tracts and scarring. Acne vulgaris (AV) is an inflammatory disorder of the pilosebaceous unit affecting adolescents and young adults. Both conditions may share common pathway leading to inflammation of the follicular unit. However, the evidence linking both the conditions is limited in strength. This study was to look for the prevalence of AV among patients with HS and also to determine the strength of the association.

This was a cross-sectional study using health system data analysis. Clinical information from the laboratories, electronic medical records, practice management systems and claims were collected and matched. The data was standardized according to common classification and vocabularies. A total of 48,085 adult patients with HS were identified. On analyzing the results, the chances of patients with HS having AV were substantially higher. Also the prevalence of AV was more in women with HS. As per this study adults with HS were 4.5 times more likely to develop AV than patients without HS.

The central features in the pathogenesis of both AV and HS include follicular obstruction, dilatation and rupture. Even the inflammation may have shared features. However, this study does not establish a temporal link or casual association between these two conditions. To conclude patients with HS have increased prevalence of AV.

Key Messages

- Patients with HS have increased prevalence of acne vulgaris
- The management strategy can target both the conditions with overlapping efficacy or with concomitant therapy.

ARTICLE 114

Association of the TNF-α Gene Promoter Polymorphisms at Nucleotide-238 and -308 with Acne Susceptibility: A Meta-analysis

Wang B, He YL. Association of the TNF-α gene promoter polymorphisms at nucleotide-238 and -308 with acne susceptibility: a meta-analysis.
Clin Exp Dermatol. 2019;44(2):176-83.

Abstract

The role of gene polymorphisms in the pathogenesis of acne has been checked in various studies. The tumor necrosis factor (TNF)-α-238 and -308 polymorphisms are considered significant genes that may serve as modulators in susceptibility to acne. This study is a meta-analysis of various case control studies to look for the association between (TNF)-α-238 and -308 polymorphisms and acne susceptibility. Different databases like PubMed, EMBASE, Scopus, SinoMed and China National Knowledge Infrastructure were searched to identify eligible studies and 95% CI were calculated to evaluate the association. A total of seven independent case control studies were finalized. The findings of this study showed a significant association between A allele of the TNF-α-238 polymorphism and susceptibility to acne in Asian population, TNF-α-308 polymorphism was associated with increased susceptibility to acne in Asian and Turkish population. However both the variations did not show the association in European population.

COMMENT

The tumor necrosis factor (TNF)-α is a significant immune response mediator. *Propionibacterium acnes* has shown to stimulate TNF-α synthesis from keratinocytes and monocytes through Toll like receptor activation and hence play a role in the pathogenesis of acne. Elevated TNF-α levels have been found in acne lesions. The gene for TNF-α is located on chromosome 6. Various single nucleotide polymorphisms have been detected in TNF-α. The commonly studied polymorphisms are at -238 and -308 of the promoted region. Multiple studies have shown association between these two single nucleotide polymorphisms (SNPs) and acne susceptibility. However owing to the different methodology, small sample size and clinical differences, the results have been contradictory rather than convincing. Hence this meta-analysis study was done to confirm the association between these polymorphisms and acne susceptibility.

A thorough search was done to identify various case control studies evaluating the role of TNF-α-238 and -308 polymorphisms with acne susceptibility. Various databases like PubMed, EMBASE, Scopus, SinoMed and China National Knowledge Infrastructure have been searched to look for eligible studies. The key words used for search included 'genetics, polymorphism, susceptibility, acne, risk, acne vulgaris and TNF-α'.

Studies were selected based on strict inclusion and exclusion criteria. Only case control association studies were considered for the analysis. Seven eligible studies were included for the meta-analysis. A total of 1053 patients with acne were evaluated in the analysis. The association of TNF-α-238 polymorphisms was evaluated in Asian and European populations. "A" allele was associated with increased acne susceptibility in Asian population but not in European population. The evaluation of TNF-α-308 polymorphism with acne susceptibility was done in Asian, European, Arab and Turkish populations. An association with acne susceptibility was found in Asian and Turkish population but not in European and Arab population. Even a meta-regression analysis was also performed to look for sources of heterogenecity and publication bias. There was no publication bias as per results of Egger test.

This literature review and meta-analysis has shown a significant association of TNF-α-238 and -308 polymorphisms with acne susceptibility in Asian and Turkish population. This has been one of the largest meta-analysis done till date with around 2203 participants. Further larger studies may be needed for a more definitive conclusion.

Key Messages

- TNF-α plays an important role in the pathogenesis of acne
- TNF-α-238 and -308 polymorphisms are associated with susceptibility to acne.

ARTICLE 115

Tumor Necrosis Factor α-308 G/A and Interleukin 1 β-511 C/T Gene Polymorphisms in Patients with Scarring Acne

Akoglu G, Tan C, Ayvaz DC, et al. Tumor necrosis factor α-308 G/A and interleukin 1 β-511 C/T gene polymorphisms in patients with scarring acne.
J Cosmet Dermatol. 2019;18(1):395-400.

Abstract

Acne is a chronic inflammatory skin disorder of the pilosebaceous unit. It may result in scarring causing psychological morbidity. The tumor necrosis factor (TNF)-α and interleukin-1 beta (IL-1β) are the proinflammatory mediators in acne pathogenesis. This study was done to look for the association between TNF-α-308 and IL-1β-511 gene polymorphisms with acne, post-acne scarring susceptibility and acne severity. The study included 90 patients with acne vulgaris and

30 healthy controls. Patients were sub-grouped on the basis of acne severity and acne scarring. Real-time PCR was done on peripheral venous samples for detecting TNF-α-308 and IL-1β-511 genotypic variants. However, there was no association found between TNF-α-308 and IL-1β-511 polymorphic variants with acne and post-acne scarring susceptibility and acne severity.

COMMENT

Acne is a chronic inflammatory disorder of pilosebaceous units affecting mainly the adolescents and young adults. Proinflammatory cytokines tumor necrosis factor-α (TNF-α) and interleukin-1 beta (IL-1β) trigger the inflammation in acne after stimulation by *Propionibacterium acnes*. Genetic factors are considered important as family history of severe acne is seen in many patients. Gene polymorphisms have been shown to increase cytokine levels and also affect the acne pathogenesis. This study is done on the hypothesis that genotypic variation in locus of TNF-α-308 and IL-1β-511 may be associated acne, acne severity, and scarring.

This was a case control study done on patients attending dermatology OPD. A total of 90 acne patients were enrolled after considering the inclusion and exclusion criteria. Thirty healthy individuals were included as controls. Acne grading was done using Global Acne Grading System. Peripheral blood samples were drawn from all patients real time PCR was done to detect TNF-α-308 and IL-1β-511 genotypic variants. Patients were classified into mild, moderate, and severe acne and also into scarring and non-scarring group. Scarring was seen in around 36 patients (30%). The distribution of genotypes of TNF-α-308 and IL-1β-511 were similar between the acne and the healthy subjects. Even in scarring and non-scarring group there was no significant change was detected.

To conclude, this was a preliminary investigation of the role of gene polymorphisms in the pathogenesis of acne and acne severity. There was no significant association detected in this study. However, further larger studies and looking for other genotypic variants may demonstrate the role in pathogenesis of acne vulgaris.

Key Messages

- *Tumor necrosis factor alpha (TNF-α) and interleukin-1 β (IL-1β) are main proinflammatory mediators of acne pathogenesis*
- *TNF-α-308 and IL-1β polymorphic variants are not associated with acne and post-acne scarring susceptibility and acne severity.*

ARTICLE 116

SIG1459: A Novel Phytyl-Cysteine Derived TLR2 Modulator with In Vitro and Clinical Anti-acne Activity

Fernández JR, Webb C, Rouzard K, et al. SIG1459: A novel phytyl-cysteine derived TLR2 modulator with in vitro and clinical antiacne activity.
Exp Dermatol. 2018;27(9):993-9.

Abstract

Cutibacterium (formerly *Propionibacterium acnes*) is an important factor in the pathogenesis of acne. Initiation of an innate immune response in keratinocytes via recognition and activation of toll-like receptor-2(TLR2) is a key step in comedogenesis. Tetramethyl-hexadecenyl-cysteine-formylprolinate (SIG1459), a novel anti-acne isoprenylcysteine (IPC) small molecule, is shown to have direct antibacterial activity and inhibit TLR2 inflammatory signaling. Results showed that 1% SIG1459 significantly outperformed 3% benzoyl peroxide (BPO) over 8 weeks, resulting in 79% improvement as compared to 56% for BPO. Also, it was well tolerated. Hence, SIG1459 and phytyl IPC compounds represent a novel anti-acne technology that provides a safe dual modulating benefit by killing *C. acnes* and reducing the inflammation it triggers via TLR2 signaling.

COMMENT

Acne is one of the most common inflammatory disorders of the pilosebaceous unit. *Cutibacterium acnes* plays an important role in the pathogenesis of acne vulgaris. Follicular hyperkeratinization and inflammation have been shown to be mediated through toll-like receptor-2 (TLR-2). The various treatment options for acne include topical and oral retinoids, antibiotics, and topical antimicrobials. However, there are chances of side effects and antimicrobial resistance while using these agents. Hence newer drugs with unique modes of action are being investigated. This study was to evaluate the in vitro and clinical anti-acne activity of SIG 1459: A novel phytyl-cysteine derived TLR2 modulator. Sixty-five patients completed the study, 30 patients received 1% SIG1459 cream, 15 received 3% benzoyl peroxide (BPO) and 15 received vehicle cream. Patients with mild-to-moderate acne were included in the study. The study duration was for 8 weeks.

Antibacterial activity against *C. acnes*: The antibacterial properties of SIG1459 was investigated by checking the minimum inhibitory concentration (MIC) and minimum bactericidal concentration (MBC) values versus two commonly available *C. acnes* strains isolated from facial acne. MIC value of SIG1459 was almost 200 times more potent than BPO and MBC was about 800 times more compared to BPO. Also it had an effect on biofilm eradication. The minimum biofilm eradication concentration of SIG1459 was better than BPO and salicylic acid.

Inhibition of TLR-2 activated cytokine release: Increased expression of TLR-2 has been seen in acne vulgaris contributing to the inflammatory response. This study shows that SIG1549 significantly inhibits *C. acnes* induced IL–8 release. Once again the efficacy was better compared to BPO and salicylic acid.

Comparison with BPO in human subjects: First SIG1459 was tested with human repeated insult patch test to look for sensitization and irritation. Followed by this 1% SIG1459 cream was studied in single blind vehicle controlled study in subjects with acne prone skin and compared with 3% BPO which is a commonly used anti-acne preparation. SIG1459 cream was well tolerated by the patients. There was a statistically significant improvement in acne in the SIG1459 group compared to 3% BPO and vehicle group. There was 77% decline in investigator global assessment score compared to baseline. Also photographs taken using UV illumination showed reduced porphyrin levels which once again confirmed the antibacterial activity of SIG1459.

To conclude SIG1459 has a strong anti-inflammatory and antibacterial activity with a good safety profile. It also has an action against TLR-2 induced cytokines. The clinical study demonstrates good efficacy compared to 3% BPO, but with minimal side effects. Further larger studies can evaluate the role of SIG1459 as a novel anti-acne preparation.

Key Messages

- *SIG1459 has significant antibacterial activity against Propionibacterium acnes*
- *SIG1459 was better than 3% BPO in both efficacy and tolerability. This could be a novel anti-acne technology.*

ARTICLE 117

Associations among Two Vitamin D Receptor (VDR) Gene Polymorphisms (ApaI and TaqI) in Acne Vulgaris: A Pilot Susceptibility Study

Swelam MM, El-Barbary RA, Saudi WM, et al. Associations among two vitamin D receptor (VDR) gene polymorphisms (ApaI and TaqI) in acne vulgaris: A pilot susceptibility study.
J Cosmet Dermatol. 2019;18(4):1113-1120.

Abstract

The pathogenesis of acne vulgaris (AV) is multifactorial. Vitamin D (Vit D) has an important role in the differentiation and functioning of sebocytes which is mediated by nuclear Vit D receptor (VDR). Many inflammatory skin diseases have been found to be associated with genetic variations in the VDR gene and receptor dysfunction. This was a case control study done in 30 acne patients attending dermatology outpatient clinic and 30 age and sex matched controls. Serum 25(OH) D was assessed in all patients and also polymorphisms in VDR gene Apal and Taql were examined using polymerase chain reaction restriction fragment length polymorphism. Compared to controls, there was significant reduction in Apal A allele and AATT combined genotype and increase in Taql tt genotype and t allele in patients. Based on these findings, Vit D deficiency can be considered a risk factor for AV development and also VDR gene polymorphisms of Apal and Taql may play a role in pathogenesis of acne.

COMMENT

Acne vulgaris is a common disorder of the pilosebaceous unit. The pathogenesis of acne is multifactorial involving excess sebum secretion, follicular hyperkeratosis, proliferation of *Propionibacterium acnes*, inflammation, and genetics.

Keratinocytes and sebocytes are considered to be vitamin D3 responsive cells. Vitamin D (Vit D) suppresses sebum secretion and also regulates the proliferation and differentiation of keratinocytes. Vit D has been reported to have a role in the pathogenesis of acne. Vit D acts through its nuclear Vit D receptor (VDR) by controlling the transcription of target genes. VDR polymorphisms have been associated with various inflammatory skin disorders.

This was a case control study done to evaluate the role of VDR gene polymorphisms in patients with acne vulgaris. The aim of the study was to assess the association between VDR Apal and Taql gene polymorphism and susceptibility to AV. The study was conducted in 30 patients with AV and 30 age and sex matched controls. Patients with history of autoimmune diseases, drugs causing acneiform eruptions, Vit D, calcium, steroid medications, hormonal imbalance, and pregnant women were excluded from the study. Two venous blood samples were taken from each participant, one for estimation of Vit D and other for detection of VDR Taql and Apal genes polymorphisms using restriction fragment length polymorphism (PCR RFLP).

Family history was positive in 19 patients. About 6, 10 and 14 patients had mild, moderate and severe acne respectively. The tt genotype and t allele were considered risky for acne development whereas Apal A allele and AATT combined genotype were considered protective against acne development. There was no statistically significant difference between AV patients and controls, with no association between acne regarding Apal, Taql, and combined genotypes. No significant differences were found between various Apal, Taql combined genotypes regarding clinical and laboratory data of patients.

Vitamin D concentrations were significantly lower in AV patients compared to controls. Also previous studies have shown that Vit D deficiency causes excess seborrhea, follicular hyperkeratinization, overgrowth of *P. acnes* and inflammation in AV. So Vit D deficiency may be risk factor for the development of AV and also patients with AV might benefit from Vit D treatment.

This is one of the first studies to evaluate the association between VDR polymorphisms Apal and Taql and acne vulgaris. Variations in VDR gene might cause VDR dysfunction affecting keratinocyte proliferation and differentiation, hence playing in a role in pathogenesis of skin diseases. Around 25 different polymorphisms have been reported within the VDR locus. However, ApaI and TaqI are commonly studied in several conditions.

In the present study, an association has been detected between the ApaI A allele and acne. An allele, AATT combined genotype, and AT haplotype were significantly less frequent in patients, hence were considered protective against acne development. Also there is significant increase in frequency of TaqI tt genotype and t allele in patients compared to controls which make them more prone to development of AV. However, further larger studies are needed to confirm the association and to detect the potential gene-environment interactions.

> **Key Messages**
> - *Vitamin D3 gene polymorphisms might be associated with pathogenesis of acne*
> - *There is increased frequency of TaqI tt genotype and t allele in patients with acne*
> - *AATT genotype and AT haplotype are less frequent in acne patients and may be protective against acne development.*

ARTICLE 118

Using Network Oriented Research Assistant (NORA) Technology to Compare Digital Photographic with In-Person Assessment of Acne Vulgaris

Singer HM, Almazan T, Craft N, et al. Using network oriented research assistant (NORA) technology to compare digital photographic with in-person assessment of acne vulgaris.
JAMA Dermatol. 2018;154(2):188-90.

Abstract

This study was done to compare patient-taken photographs of acne using Network Oriented Research Assistant (NORA) and Investigator's Global Assessment (IGA) findings with in-person examination findings.

This was a pilot reliability study conducted in patients with acne vulgaris from a single general dermatology clinic in Los Angeles, California, who could use NORA on an iPhone 6 to take self-photographs. Each individual underwent in-person and digital evaluation of his/her acne by the same dermatologist. All the patients were instructed on how to use NORA on the phone and also to take photographs. A total of 69 patients were enrolled in the study. It showed a strong agreement in the intraclass correlation coefficients of in-person and photograph based acne evaluations. To conclude, NORA can be used in teledermatology for research and hence to increase access to dermatology care.

COMMENT

Teledermatology has been used since many years which help to ease access to specialist care and augment traditional face-to-face consultations. However, considering the exponential growth in this field, it is necessary to ensure the validity, safety of feasibility of these applications. The main aim of this study was to determine the accuracy and reliability of acne scoring through digital photographs taken by patients on iPhone using Network Oriented Research Assistant (NORA) compared to in-person examination findings.

Investigator's Global Assessment (range 0–5, higher score indicates more severity) and lesion counting were used in standardized clinical research acne severity scoring. A total of 69 patients were included in the study. The first 9 patients were used for prototyping the workflow and photography. A total of 60 patients were evaluated by a dermatologist and also through digital self-taken photographs using NORA. There was a gap of one week between the two evaluations. The results demonstrate that the IGA and lesion counts can be reliably assessed using patient taken digital photographs with NORA.

Hence use of NORA platform in telemedicine-based clinical trial can increased accessibility, diversity of patients and improved adherence among patients to the study.

Key Messages
- There has been an agreement between evaluations performed in person and from self-photographs taken using NORA
- The NORA platform on mobile devices can be used for evaluation in telemedicine-based clinical trials on acne.

ARTICLE 119

Genetic Association between the *NLRP3* Gene and Acne Vulgaris in a Chinese Population

Shen C, Wang QZ, Shen ZY, et al. Genetic Association between the *NLRP3* Gene and Acne Vulgaris in a Chinese Population.
Clin Exp Dermatol. 2019;44(2):184-9.

Abstract
Acne vulgaris (AV) is a common chronic inflammatory skin disease. There are reports to suggest that inflammasomes play an important role in infection and immunity of AV. The activation of

innate immune system relies on a family of receptors called pattern recognition receptors (PRRs). The PRR family includes NLRP3, which is capable of forming NLRP3 inflammasome. The present study, conducted on Chinese population, showed us that the rs10754558 of NLRP3 is associated with acne susceptibility.

COMMENT

Acne vulgaris (AV) is a common chronic inflammatory skin disease of the sebaceous glands. Inflammation plays an important role in the pathogenesis of acne. The role of genetic factors in the pathogenesis of acne has been demonstrated by family and twin studies, though the underlying genetic basis remains unclear. *Propionibacterium acnes* (*P. acnes*) plays an important role in the pathogenesis of acne by activating innate immune system. The activation of innate immune system relies on a family of receptors called pattern recognition receptors (PRRs). The PRR family includes NLRP3, which is capable of forming NLRP3 inflammasome. A group of bacterial toxins, the pathogen-associated molecular pattern molecules (PAMPs), and the damage-associated molecular pattern molecules (DAMPs) activate NLRP3 inflammasome, which further leads to induction of signal activations including Ca^{2+} signaling, generation of reactive oxygen species (ROS), and K^+ efflux and lysosomal rupture.

There are reports of NLRP3 polymorphisms being involved in the mediation and occurrence of inflammation. The various genetic studies involving NLRP3 polymorphisms have supported the role of NLRP3 in other inflammatory diseases, such as type 2 diabetes mellitus (T2DM), rheumatoid arthritis, and atherosclerosis.

There are reports to suggest that inflammasomes play an important role in infection and immunity of AV. However, only a few studies have been reported on NLRP3 and acne vulgaris. The present study was undertaken to investigate two single nucleotide polymorphisms (SNPs) in the *NLRP3* gene in patients with AV and healthy controls (HCs) in a Chinese population. The present case-control study was conducted with 428 patients with AV and 384 HCs.

Genotyping of two SNPs, rs10754558, and rs4612666 of the *NLRP3* gene was done using polymerase chain reaction (PCR) with sequence-specific primers. To ascertain whether the SNP rs10754558 might be responsible for the altered *NLRP3* gene expression in AV by disrupting the interaction between micro-RNA (miR)-4273 and NLRP3 mRNA, a dual luciferase reporter assay was performed. The mRNA level of NLRP3 in both the groups was measured by PCR. The frequencies of the G allele of rs10754558 were 0.54 and 0.49 in patients with acne vulgaris and HCs respectively ($p < 0.05$), whereas no significant difference was observed for SNP rs4612666.

When dual luciferase reporter assay was performed, it was found that luciferase activity was downregulated by about 40% when the G allele of rs10754558 coexisted with miRNA-4273. The above finding indicates that the G allele might interfere with miR-4273 function and alter NLRP3 expression. The comparison of the level of NLRP3 mRNA among both the groups revealed that patients with AV had a significantly higher level than that in HCs.

In recent past, there have been three studies that have attempted to reveal the mechanism, which regulates these inflammatory responses partially via an NLRP3-mediated pathway. In a study conducted by Qin et al. it was found that human monocytes respond to *P. acnes* and secrete mature interleukin-1 β (IL-β), and live *P. acnes* that stimulates monocytes cause upregulation of expression of the caspase-1 gene within the monocytes. A rodent model analyzed by Li et al. found that IL-1β mRNA was upregulated and NLRP3 inflammasomes were activated in the inflammatory acne lesions. Li et al. also suggested that neutrophilic inflammatory lesions were triggered by NLRP3 inflammasomes and IL-1β and may be contributed to *P. acnes*-associated inflammation in vivo.

The study done by Kistowska et al. reported that *P. acnes* triggers monocyte–macrophage NLRP3 inflammasome activation and IL-1β processing and secretion. The above findings are also true in PAPA (pyogenic arthritis, pyoderma gangrenosum and acne) syndrome in which proinflammatory cytokines and chemokines activate caspase-1 and overproduction of IL-1β, these in turn recruit and activate neutrophils, resulting in neutrophil-mediated inflammation.

The SNP rs10754558 is involved in the stability and expression of mRNA. A person's susceptibility to disorders, such as metabolic diseases (aspirin-induced asthma), infectious diseases (human immunodeficiency virus infection), and autoimmune diseases (T1DM and insulin resistance with T2DM), is altered by SNPs. All these studies have reported that rs10754558 SNP might be associated with the innate immune receptor of NLRP3.

The present study showed us that in the study population, the rs10754558 of NLRP3 is associated with acne susceptibility. The rs10754558 of NLRP3 might be a genetic variant of the immune systems, as the frequencies of G allele of the rs10754558 were found to be significantly higher in patients with AV than HCs.

Key Messages

- In the present study, the G allele of rs10754558 in NLRP3 is high in patients with acne vulgaris compared to healthy controls
- The NLRP3 mRNA levels are significantly higher in patients with acne than in healthy controls.

ARTICLE 120

Serum Irisin: A Prognostic Marker for Severe Acne Vulgaris

Mustafa AI, El-Shimi OS. Serum irisin: A prognostic marker for severe acne vulgaris.
J Cosmet Dermatol. 2018;17(5):931-4.

Abstract

Acne vulgaris (AV) is a chronic inflammatory disorder involving pilosebaceous units. Irisin, an adipokine, may play a role in acne vulgaris and insulin resistance. This study found that the level of serum irisin was significantly lower in AV patients than in control group, with the increase in severity of acne, irisin decreased significantly. A negative correlation was seen between serum irisin and insulin resistance among patients with acne. Irisin may act as an indicator for severity of acne.

COMMENT

Acne vulgaris is a common chronic inflammatory skin disease involving pilosebaceous units. Adipokines are secreted by adipose tissue and function as signaling networks communicating it with different organs. Adipokines may play a role in pathogenesis of acne vulgaris, and insulin resistance. Irisin is a hormone-like myokine and is one of the adipokines. Irisin is secreted mainly by adipose tissue and muscles, so it acts as an exercise-induced insulin sensitizer.

Anthropometric and biochemical parameters, hormones and adipokines, obesity, insulin resistance, type 2 diabetes mellitus (T2DM), and metabolic syndrome have all found to be associated with irisin. Irisin protects against obesity and insulin resistance by acting on subcutaneous adipose tissue, thereby increasing thermogenesis and energy expenditure. Irisin has anti-inflammatory, antioxidant, and antidiabetic effects.

The study was conducted with an aim to evaluate serum irisin levels in patients with acne vulgaris in order to assess its role along with insulin resistance in the pathogenesis of acne and severity. Sixty patients with acne vulgaris, and sixty apparently healthy controls underwent measurement of serum irisin levels by ELISA (enzyme-linked immunosorbent assay) technique. The Homeostasis Model Assessment of Insulin Resistance (HOMA-IR) index was used to calculate insulin resistance.

The level of serum irisin was significantly lower in acne vulgaris patients than in control group ($p < 0.001$). A negative correlation was seen between serum irisin and insulin resistance among patients. It was also noted that with the increase in severity of acne, irisin decreased significantly. Inflammation is one the important factors in the pathogenesis of acne vulgaris. Studies have shown that adipogenic factors, galectin-12, resistin, stearoyl-CoA desaturase (SCD), sterol response element binding protein-1 (SREBP-1), and CCAAT–enhancer-binding protein α (C/EBPα) are expressed by both sebocytes and adipocytes during their differentiation. Hyperandrogenemia and hyperinsulinemia are among various other factors involved in causing acne vulgaris. An increase in sebaceous glands' size, sebum production and induction of keratinocyte proliferation are caused by androgens. During puberty, hyperinsulinemia may occur due to physiologic insulin resistance, thereby increasing androgen synthesis. Hyperinsulinemia causes an increase in free insulin-like growth factor-1 (IGF-1) and decreases IGF-binding protein 3, thereby resulting in acne. The IGF-1 stimulates sebocyte proliferation by increasing the mean facial sebum excretion rate, serum dihydrotestosterone, and dehydroepiandrosterone sulfate levels. Hyperinsulinemia causes an increase in epidermal growth factors and transforming growth factor-β levels, which leads to an elevated plasma nonesterified fatty acids levels, resulting in inflammation and acne.

The reduced responsiveness of target cells to insulin is seen in insulin resistance. Insulin resistance is manifested on the skin as acrochordons, acanthosis nigricans, androgenetic alopecia, acne, and hirsutism. The major factor underlying the pathogenesis of the metabolic syndrome is insulin resistance. The association between acne vulgaris, insulin resistance, and metabolic syndrome has been suggested. In the present study, it was found that patients with acne vulgaris showed significant insulin resistance than control subjects, their HOMA-IR indices showed a significant increase with the increase in severity of acne lesions. The above findings confirm the association between insulin resistance with acne vulgaris and its severity. The findings of the present study are similar to the study by Emiroğlu et al. who found the correlation between insulin resistance and severe acne vulgaris. However, studies done in postadolescent males showed a significant association between insulin resistance and acne vulgaris but there was no correlation with disease severity. Balta et al. conducted a study on adult patients, and did not find any association between insulin resistance and acne vulgaris.

Earlier studies have shown significantly lower levels of serum irisin in T2DM compared to controls. These results are similar to the negative correlation that have found in the present study between serum irisin level and insulin resistance among patients with acne vulgaris, as insulin resistance leads to diabetes mellitus. This is in favor of the findings of the present study as serum irisin level was higher in controls due to its anti-inflammatory role through reduction in both the expression and release of the proinflammatory cytokines.

This study showed that lower serum irisin and high HOMA-IR index serve as good prognostic markers for detecting the severity of acne lesions, with a significant sensitivity (88.9% and 77.8%, respectively) and specificity (76.2% and 81%, respectively). However, Chen et al. have reviewed various published studies with conflicting results about the role and effect of irisin on insulin resistance and glucose homeostasis. Thus, there is a need to elicit the role to irisin in various metabolic disorders.

Key Messages

- The level of serum irisin was significantly lower in acne vulgaris patients than in control group, with the increase in severity of acne, irisin decreased significantly
- A negative correlation was seen between serum irisin and insulin resistance among patients with acne vulgaris.

ARTICLE 121

Primary Sebocytes and Sebaceous Gland Cell Lines for Studying Sebaceous Lipogenesis and Sebaceous Gland Diseases

Schneider MR, Zouboulis CC. Primary sebocytes and sebaceous gland cell lines for studying sebaceous lipogenesis and sebaceous gland diseases.
Exp Dermatol. 2018;27(5):484-8.

Abstract

Altered sebaceous gland (SG) functions are contributory to the pathogenesis of various human skin diseases. An increased and/or modified sebum is an important feature in acne vulgaris. The degeneration of SGs is characteristic of some forms of alopecia. This article focuses on previous studies done regarding the isolation and culture of primary human sebocytes and immortalized SG cell lines; and also assessment of their contribution for the study of SGs and sebum function in skin health and disease has been done.

COMMENT

The pathogenesis of acne vulgaris and some forms of alopecia involves alteration in the sebum secretion and/or changes in the structure of SGs. The analysis of recent work on primary sebocytes and SG cell line has been done, and their contribution for better understanding of sebaceous lipogenesis and the role of the same in healthy skin and disease have been assessed.

Sebum produced by the SGs has been known to have many functions including antimicrobial and antioxidative properties. In recent past, it has shown that sebaceous lipids have known to be distributed by the SGs in their dermal periphery and to influence the activity of perifollicular macrophages. This adds the possibility of new functions to the already reported ones. Altered SG functions are contributory to the pathogenesis of various human skin diseases. An increased and/or modified sebum is an important feature in acne vulgaris. The degeneration of SG is characteristic of psoriatic alopecia and is also found in hidradenitis suppurativa, lichen planopilaris, pseudopelade of Brocq, and in some rare forms of cicatricial alopecia, such as primary cicatricial alopecia, linear morphea, and Zouboulis syndrome. A well-studied animal model for primary cicatricial alopecia is the asebia mouse, which develops SG atrophy due to a spontaneous mutation in the gene encoding the enzyme stearoyl-coenzyme A desaturase 1. Other models use rat preputial sebocytes and hamster sebocytes. The sebum composition, SG structure, and sebaceous markers are species-specific. Keratin 7 and MUC1 are sebaceous markers in human but not in murine SGs. This explains the restriction of acne to human sebaceous follicles.

The article focuses on previous studies done regarding the isolation and culture of primary human sebocytes and immortalized SG cell lines, and also assessment of their contribution for the study of SG and sebum function in skin health and disease. Xia and colleagues, in 1989, isolated SGs via microdissection from human pilosebaceous units, removed the ducts, and seeded the gland lobules on a 3T3 feeder cell layer; this was the first report in detail on the isolation, characterization, and maintenance of human sebocytes in vitro. The pilosebaceous units separated from the dermis together with the epidermis by dispase treatment. Doran and colleagues enzymatically treated to dissociate the cells and cultured on a 3T3 feeder layer. Fujie and colleagues mechanically isolated the SGs that remained attached to the epidermis after removal of the dermis, and isolated cells either by explant culture or by SG enzymatic dissociation without using a feeder layer. Researches isolated cells that exhibited expression of typical sebocyte markers, such as the epithelial membrane antigen (EMA). The ability to accumulate cytoplasmic lipid droplets upon a corresponding stimulus was also demonstrated. Zouboulis and colleagues were the first to immortalize human SG cell line, SZ95. Facial sebocytes of an 87-year-old woman were isolated and transfected with simian virus 40 large T antigen. These SZ95 sebocytes express keratin 7 and EMA, and accumulate cytoplasmic lipid droplets. They also synthesize squalene and wax esters, and respond to androgens and retinoids. The periauricular area of a 55-year-old man was used by Thiboutot and colleagues to establish the sebocyte cell line, SEB-1. The SG cells were transfected with HPV-16 E6 and E7 genes to form two immortalized human SG cell lines, SEB-E6E7 and SEBO662.

The various SG cell lines could not achieve holocrine secretion; however, they could address diverse lipogenesis and innate immunity. The sebocytes form spheroids with basement membrane when maintained in 3D culture. These, on exposure to prostaglandin E2, became larger and the organization became more complex, by activating the canonical Wnt signaling pathway as well as increasing cell viability and proliferation, mitochondrial metabolism, and lipid synthesis. A coculture of explants skin and SZ95 resulted in better structural integrity of the epidermis, higher percentage of proliferating basal cells and reduced apoptosis of differentiating epidermal cells, and SZ95 sebocytes exhibited morphological and biochemical signs of normal differentiation. The above data provides evidence about the benefits of interaction between sebocytes and skin explants, and a rationale for the integration of sebocytes in 3D skin models. The above mentioned features make SG cell lines easy-to-study molecular and cellular processes underlying sebaceous lipogenesis and their alteration in SG diseases.

In the recent times, immortalized human SG cell lines have been used to analyze sebocyte adipokines, to identify micro-RNAs associated with sebaceous differentiation, and to study the proteins associated with cytoplasmic SG lipid droplets or those secreted by sebocytes in addition to the lipid synthesized.

> **Key Messages**
> - The various immortalized SG cell lines are SZ95, SEB-1, SEB-E6E7, and SEBO662
> - The immortalized human SG cell lines have been used to analyze sebocyte adipokines, to identify micro-RNAs associated with sebaceous differentiation, and to study the proteins associated with cytoplasmic SG lipid droplets or those secreted by sebocytes in addition to the lipid synthesized.

ARTICLE 122

Acne Vulgaris in Patients with Hidradenitis Suppurativa

Ravn Jørgensen AH, Ring HC, Thomsen SF. Acne vulgaris in patients with hidradenitis suppurativa.
J Am Acad Dermatol. 2019;80(5):e129-30.

Abstract

Consecutively referred patients with hidradenitis suppurativa (HS) were analyzed for prevalence of acne vulgaris (AV) and variables were compared between patients of HS with AV and without AV. When both the groups were compared, patients of HS with AV had a lower mean age and lower age at onset of HS. There was no difference in Hurley stage in HS patients with and without AV on statistical analysis. On comparison between the groups, the levels of plasma inflammatory markers were found to be lower in HS patients with AV.

COMMENT

Wertenteil et al. conducted a study in a population-based sample from the US, found that AV among patients with HS is 15.2% compared to 2.9% for adults without HS. On further analysis, prevalence was higher among females aged 18–44 years, non-whites, obese, and patients who had polycystic ovarian syndrome (PCOS).

This study, conducted in a tertiary dermatological referral center, included consecutive newly referred patients with HS and analyzed for the prevalence of AV. The age at onset of HS, family history of HS, smoking status, diagnosis of PCOS, and race were documented and analyzed. The body mass index (BMI), Hurley score, Dermatology Life Quality Index (DLQI), anatomic region of HS, number of boils in the past month, and plasma inflammatory markers were also recorded. The study was conducted between January 1st, 2016 and October 8th, 2018. Out of the 302 patients included in the study, 191 were women and 111 men, and the mean age was 39.4 years. The prevalence of AV was 21.2%, with 19 (29.7%), 39 (60.9%), and 6 (9.4%) patients were in Hurley stage I, II, and

III, respectively. There was no difference in Hurley stage in HS patients with and without AV on statistical analysis. The patients of HS with AV had a lower mean age (33.8 vs. 40.8 years; p <0.001) and lower age at onset of HS (21.4 vs. 27.2 years; p <0.001) compared with patients of HS without AV.

The levels of plasma inflammatory markers, C-reactive protein (CRP), neutrophils, and neutrophil/lymphocyte ratio (NLR) were found to be lower in HS patients with AV compared to HS patients without AV. No statistically significant difference was observed in AV among male and female patients, smokers and non-smokers, patients with a diagnosis of PCOS, and obese and nonobese patients. No difference in DLQI score was seen among both the groups.

The findings of this study are comparable to the study by Wertenteil et al. which showed that patients with HS referred for specialized hospital care had a high prevalence of AV. There needs to be a greater awareness of the association between HS and AV, and co-management approaches can be planned for both the conditions.

Key Messages

- In this study, the patients of HS with AV had a lower mean age and lower age at onset of HS compared with patients of HS without AV
- The awareness of the association between HS and AV can help to formulate co-management approaches for both the conditions.

ARTICLE 123

Validation of 3D Skin Imaging for Objective Repeatable Quantification of Severity of Atrophic Acne Scarring

Petit L, Zugaj D, Bettoli V, et al. Validation of 3D skin imaging for objective repeatable quantification of severity of atrophic acne scarring.
Skin Res Technol. 2018;24(4):542-50.

Abstract

Atrophic scarring is one of the major sequelae of acne and present in up to 43% of acne patients. The depth and/or volume of atrophic acne scars cannot be assessed clinically and objective tools, to assess scars, are lacking. The aim of this study was to define and evaluate parameters of 3D imaging. The comparison of data showed excellent repeatability, good correlation to clinical severity, and statistically correlated with clinical observations of scars in the range of 2–4 mm.

COMMENT

Atrophic scarring is one of the major sequelae of acne and present in up to 43% of acne patients. Scarring occurs in predisposed individuals with acne as a result of acne-associated inflammation. The inflammation gets prolonged and there is inadequate wound healing, resulting in scars. Not only the scars are displeasing, but they can also be a cause of psychological distress. If there is increased repairing tissue, the scars are called hypertrophic, and if it decreased, the scars are called atrophic. Based on the shape, atrophic acne scars are further categorized into rolling, boxcar, and ice-pick scars; atrophic scars can also be categorized based on their size.

The depth and/or volume of atrophic acne scars cannot be assessed clinically and objective tools, to assess scars, are lacking. Lighting and shadows affect standard 2D photography. The study was carried out with an aim to define and evaluate parameters of 3D imaging that can be used in the assessment of atrophic acne scarring. The assessment of acne scars is difficult and partly attributed to the irregular borders and contours of skin scarring; the problem of assessment gets magnified when there are multiple scars, which is typically the case. The different imaging technologies such as stereovision, fringe interference, and advanced optical technologies used various imaging systems, which quantitatively measure skin roughness, wrinkles, and nodule formation. They can also track changes over time, and are used for microstructure skin analysis.

The aim of this study was to define and evaluate parameters of 3D imaging. The study was done in a single center and consisted of 31 patients with acne scarring. Atrophic acne scars following an acne lesion with loss of tissue (greater than normal pore diameter) were assessed. Five dermatologists evaluated the scars by the global severity of atrophic acne scarring on a 0-4 scale (clear, almost clear, mild, moderate and severe). The scars were counted and based on size they were categorized (scars <2 mm, 2-4 mm and >4 mm in diameter).

The target area was captured by three-dimensional imaging by the LifeViz Micro® system. This device is easy to use, fast and portable. Three-dimensional images are produced by combining standard photography with stereovision technology. The quantification of various skin parameters such as volume, height, depth, surface, perimeter, and roughness is done by the system using an analysis module. MountainsMaps® software was used to analyze the captured images and metrology software (Digital Surf Surface Intelligence, Besançon, France) for image analysis.

Based on ISO 21758 standard for 3D surface texture as described by Blateyron, the 3D parameters were tested, which included Valley void volumes Vvv (80%), Vvv (95%), void volume Vvv (10%), with pre- or postmorphology filtering. The parameters correspond to the volumes of the negative valley (scars). The comparison of data from V1 to V2 was excellent with an intraclass correlation (ICC) of 0.98, demonstrating Vvv had excellent repeatability. The Vvv had good correlation to clinical severity and statistically correlated with clinical observations of scars in the range of 2-4 mm. The Vvv parameter when correlated with mean global severity at the target area rating showed a correlation coefficient of 0.77. The Vvv parameter, which evaluated the volume of scars, was mainly impacted by scars >2 mm.

Brauer et al. reported that 3D imaging measurements of scar volume showed improvement with pulsed laser in scar volume by 24.3%; however, the methodology for computation of volume was not detailed and they noted a potential lack of reproducibility, which can be possibly due to variation in angle or pressure. Since LifeViz captures images without any skin contact, the problem of pressure was not encountered in this study, but the issue of alignment variation persisted even in the present study. The presence of active acne did not have a marked impact on reproducibility of scar assessment, and it is an advantage of this technology.

Key Messages

- On 3D imaging and analysis, the parameter, Vvv (volume of scars mm2), had excellent repeatability, good correlation to clinical severity, and statistically correlated with clinical observations of scars in the range of 2–4 mm
- The presence of active acne lesions did not have a marked impact on reproducibility of scar assessment, and it is an advantage of this technology.

ARTICLE 124

No Evidence for Follicular Keratinocyte Hyperproliferation in Acne Lesions as Compared to Autologous Healthy Hair Follicles

Persson G, Johansson-Jänkänpää E, Ganceviciene R, et al. No evidence for follicular keratinocyte hyperproliferation in acne lesions as compared to autologous healthy hair follicles.
Exp Dermatol. 2018;27(6):668-71.

Abstract

The sebaceous hair follicles with abnormal hyperkeratinization have been believed to play a role in the pathogenesis of acne. This study was conducted to get a better insight into hyperkeratinization by measuring the expression of proliferation, mitosis, and apoptosis markers.

The levels of Ki67, α-tubulin, phosphohistone H3, and cleaved-PARP were measured. The study findings revealed that there was no increase in keratinocyte proliferation in acne vulgaris, further studies are required to understand the alternative mechanisms, which are responsible for infundibular hyperkeratinization.

COMMENT

Abnormalities in the production of sebum, sebocyte differentiation, proliferation, and inflammation are thought to contribute to the development of acne. Approximately around 200,000 hair follicles are present on the scalp with around 5,000 hair follicles on the face, and at any given point, less than 1% of the follicles are affected. Although, sebum and hormonal dysregulation may be needed to cause acne, there must be a local mechanism, which affects a tiny number of hair follicles. Abnormal hyperproliferation in the infundibulum of the hair follicle has been thought to play a role in acne, with various studies reporting a higher expression of Ki67, keratin 6, 16, and 17, and psoriasin (S100A7), which is a member of the *S100* gene family in acne lesions.

Taking into account the drawbacks of the previous studies such as low number of enrolled patients and anatomically unmatched controls, larger number of patients and age-matched controls were enrolled in the study. Ki67, which is an objective measure of proliferation, was counted only in the epidermis and the basal layer of epidermis and hair follicles, which suggested that affinity of the antibodies used was very low, and hence the lowered sensitivity of the applied methods.

The evaluation of Ki67, K16, and p63 demonstrated that acne affected hair follicles and the controls show a similar proliferation status, which is not in favor of earlier reports. A fine balance between cell proliferation and apoptosis is required for keratinocyte development, which are both regulated by cell cycle regulators. The above process is required for formation of stratum corneum and skin appendages including pilosebaceous units. The other two proliferative markers that were measured in this study were phosphorylated histone H3 (phosphohistone H3) and α-tubulin. An apoptotic marker, cleaved poly (ADP-ribose) polymerase (cleaved-PARP), was also measured.

The cohort consisted of 66 patients with acne, 40 males and 26 females. The median age of the cohort population was 22 years (range was 15–45 years). Out of the biopsies from acne lesions, 60 were from the back and 6 from face, with 31 acne papules, 28 pustules, 6 nodules, and 1 cyst. About 12 biopsies were taken from macroscopically unaffected skin in the same area as that of acne biopsy, 7 were from the back and 5 were from the face.

The assessment of Ki67 was done using immunohistochemistry. Immunofluorescence microscopy was used to assess a-tubulin, phosphohistone H3, and cleaved-PARP. The α-tubulin staining was universal, and there was no change in assembly. The expression of α-tubulin was considered as a marker of preserved quality, which reflected the anatomical integrity of biopsy specimens. When the expression of cleaved-PARP was measured, it was seen to be a rare. The cell proliferation rate was measured by the expression of Ki67 and phosphohistone H3, and was found to be similar between acne and the two control groups.

On further investigation, there was no significant difference in the keratinocyte proliferation in pustules or nodules. This study shows that there is no increased keratinocyte proliferation in acne vulgaris, suggesting the role of alternative mechanisms that might result in infundibular hyperkeratinization in acne.

> **Key Messages**
>
> - The measurement of proliferative markers Ki67, a-tubulin, and phosphohistone H3, and an apoptotic marker, cleaved-PARP, which reflect abnormal hyperkeratinization in the sebaceous follicles, were similar in patients with acne and controls
> - Alternative mechanisms that might result in infundibular hyperkeratinization in acne should be investigated.

ARTICLE 125

Seasonal Changes in Epidermal Ceramides are Linked to Impaired Barrier Function in Acne Patients

Pappas A, Kendall AC, Brownbridge LC, et al. Seasonal changes in epidermal ceramides are linked to impaired barrier function in acne patients.
Exp Dermatol. 2018;27(8):833-6.

Abstract

Recent literature shows that reduced epidermal barrier function has a role in acne, with worsening of the symptoms in summer. An impairment of barrier function correlates with reduction in total sphingolipids; however, there is lack of detailed understanding of stratum corneum (SC) ceramide (CER) changes and their role in barrier function in the disease. In healthy individuals, a seasonal variation in SC ceramides is present, where acylceramides CER(EOS) are found to be reduced in winter, but the role in acne is not clear.

COMMENT

The study was done to compare acne with healthy skin, to find out the potential seasonal differences by interrogation, and to analyze any association with barrier function. A detailed investigation of stratum corneum (SC) ceramides was done throughout the year. Seven adolescent males with acne and 10 without acne aged between 13 years and 18 years were included in the study. The study subjects had acne over 12 months and females were excluded to avoid the effect of hormonal cycling effect.

The samples were taken using Leukoflex® tapes from cheeks for analysis of SC lipids in February, April, August and November to cover all the seasons. Each donor was analyzed using a single tape-strip to extract the ceramides. Identification and analysis were done by ultra-performance-liquid-chromatography coupled to electrosprayionization tandem mass-spectrometry (UPLC/ESI-MS/MS) resulting in 238 ceramides from 10 classes. The ceramide, CER[N(25)S(18)], found in negligible levels endogenously was used as internal standard and also for relative semiquantitation.

The proportion of ceramide classes (mean % of total ceramides) was similar to previous analysis of cheek SC. The samples taken from cheek had CER(AH) and CER(NH) abundantly, while the body sites such as forearm had different composition, less 6-hydroxy-ceramides and more phytoceramides.

Transepidermal water loss (TEWL) assessed by open-chambered evaporimeter revealed that acne-affected skin had a higher value compared to healthy skin throughout the year. This could possibly indicate a compromised barrier function. Acne symptoms were assessed using modified Cook's score and did not show any seasonal change. A significant negative correlation was observed between ceramide classes and TEWL, but only some between ceramide classes and acne symptoms. The TEWL did not show any correlation with symptoms and so ceramide class totals in healthy and acne skin were compared.

Lower levels of ceramides, i.e. CER(NH) (February: 57% $p = 0.004$; April: 38% $p = 0.001$), CER(AH) (February: 36% $p = 0.003$; April: 47% $p = 0.006$), CER(EOS) (February: 68% $p <0.0001$; August: 71% $p = 0.003$; November: 40% $p = 0.002$), and CER(EOH) (February: 59% $p = 0.006$), were noted. The differences in ceramides equilibrated in August, probably when the TEWL differences diminished. This suggests that changes in the barrier function may be not only due to differential ceramide production in acne, but also due to reduced levels of CER(NH) and CER(AH) species.

The CER(NH) and CER(AH) species were low in acne compared with healthy skin, and CER(EOS) and CER(EOH) species with 18-carbon sphingoid bases were also found to be in reduced levels. Thus, this study reveals that seasonal variations in skin ceramides are more evident in acne skin, with the reductions in ceramide levels during winter months. During winter months, there is reduced barrier function, which is assessed by an increase in TEWL. Higher levels of CER(NH) and CER(AH) are produced by healthy skin in winter suggesting adaptation to temperature, humidity, or UV changes, whereas acne-affected skin is less able to do the same. At present, the mechanisms underlying seasonal changes in skin ceramides are not understood, but could possibly be due to both the ceramide salvage and de novo biosynthesis pathways.

The levels of CER(EOS) and CER(EOH) levels are crucial for SC organization and barrier function, but there seems to be very little understanding of the properties of 6-hydroxy-ceramides CER(AH) and CER(NH). The model membranes which had CER(NH) instead of CER(NS) demonstrated reduced ion permeability, although this was accompanied by increased water permeability. The lipid packing is altered by the presence of multiple hydroxyl groups [three in CER(NH), four in CER(AH)], which is similar to inclusion of phytoceramides in model membranes. The physiological significance of the above findings remains unclear, and probably implies that an effective barrier is formed by the inclusion of correct proportions of different ceramide classes.

The ceramide species found to be low in acne are all derived from the H18 sphingoid base that contains nonhydroxy (N) and α-hydroxy (A) acyl chains with

24- and 26-carbons, they are CER[(N(24)H(18)], CER[N(26)H(18)], CER[A(24)H(18)], and CER[A(26)H(18)]. This could be due to abundance of 8-carbon chains. However, the biosynthetic reactions regulating these hydroxylated ceramides are unclear.

This study brings across that changes in ceramide composition are associated with acne. Further, studies need to be conducted for better understanding of the role of ceramides and their seasonal variation leading to impaired barrier function in acne.

Key Messages

- Lower levels of ceramides were found in acne-affected skin with a notable reduction in CER(NH) and CER(AH]) as well as acylceramides, CER(EOS) and CER(EOH), and the differences were more marked in the winter months
- When compared with healthy skin, lower ceramide levels with increased TEWL were seen in skin of patients with acne, and it partly resolves in summer.

ARTICLE 126

Cutibacterium acnes (Propionibacterium acnes) and Acne Vulgaris: A Brief Look at the Latest Updates

Dréno B, Pécastaings S, Corvec S, et al. *Cutibacterium acnes (Propionibacterium acnes) and acne vulgaris: a brief look at the latest updates.*
J Eur Acad Dermatol Venereol. 2018;32 Suppl 2:5-14.

Abstract

Propionibacterium acnes (P. acnes) is a commensal bacterium, which can act as a pathogen in acne vulgaris. Patients with acne vulgaris do not have more *P. acnes* in the follicles when compared to patients with no acne. The loss of the diverse microbes along with activation of innate immunity may lead to the chronic inflammation seen in acne. The new taxonomic classification of *P. acnes* renamed as *Cutibacterium acnes (C. acnes)*, along with characterization of its phylogenetic cluster groups, has been presented here.

COMMENT

Propionibacterium acnes/Cutibacterium acnes is a gram-positive anaerobic bacterium belonging to the Actinobacteria phylum. *P. acnes/C. acnes* resides predominantly deep within the lipid-rich sebaceous follicles where they are in contact with the keratinocytes and protect skin from other harmful pathogens to preserve the stability of resident skin microbes. However, on the skin surface, they represent <2% of all bacteria, whereas *Staphylococcus epidermidis* (*S. epidermidis*) populates with >27% of the total bacteria. Intestine, stomach, lungs, mouth, conjunctiva, prostate and urinary tract are other tissues where *P. acnes/C. acnes* is found.

Short-chain fatty acids, including propionic acid, are released after degradation of sebum by *P. acnes/C. acnes*, which maintain an acidic skin pH. Recent investigations including a high-resolution core genome analysis combining *16S rRNA* gene sequences, DNA G+C content, genome size and genes content have ascertained the phylogeny of the Propionibacteriaceae family. This is an attempt to understand how species relate to each other and decode the adaptive processes involved in the transmission and evolutionary adaptation of *P. acnes* to human skin.

Identification of specific genes, such as lipase genes encoding for triacylglycerol lipase and lysophospholipase able to specifically degrade sebum lipids (whereas others were lost by deletions as a part of the evolutionary adaptation) of cutaneous *Propionibacterium* to human skin, led to definition of a new genus for cutaneous bacteria, the genus *Cutibacterium gen. nov*, which accommodates the former cutaneous species. *Propionibacterium acnes* was renamed *C. acnes* accounting for the taxonomic reclassification and for all the genomic adaptive changes. Renaming was done to differentiate it from other environmental *Propionibacterium* species, including those present in dairy products and cattle rumen.

Advanced genomic techniques and/or new sampling methods in the recent times have shown that *C. acnes* is the most predominant bacterium of pilosebaceous follicles both in acne patients and in individuals with unaffected skin. This has led to the hypothesis that some strains may be truly commensal and contribute to skin health, and others might act as pathogens.

Proteomic analysis of *C. acnes* phylotypes (IA1, IA2, IB1, IB2, II and III) revealed differently expressed proteins including adhesion proteins, CAMP factors, and one cell surface hydrolase. Further, on analysis, *C. acnes* phylotypes were classified according to their proinflammatory potential from the strongest to the mildest—type III, II, IC, IA1 and IB.

Other than virulence factors, various genes on the *C. acnes* genome that encode for glycosyltransferase, uridine diphosphate-N-acetylglucosamine-2-epimerase, and polysaccharide biosynthesis proteins are actively involved in the formation of biofilm, which plays a role in the pathophysiology of acne. Sessile *C. acnes* cells, which grow in biofilms, are more resistant to traditional antimicrobial agents compared to planktonic (free) cells, even if antibiotic-sensitive strains are present in the biofilm. Sessile *C. acnes* has a greater extracellular lipase activity, which is known to play a role in inflammation.

It is known that *Propionibacterium* species are resistant to 5-nitroimidazole agents, aminoglycosides, sulfonamides, and mupirocin; and *C. acnes* is susceptible to a wide variety of antimicrobials. Resistance of *C. acnes* to antibiotics has gradually emerged over the years and poses a problem worldwide. The chromosomal point mutations, mainly in the *23S rRNA* gene for macrolides resistance and *16S rRNA* gene for tetracycline resistance, are the most common mechanisms of antibiotic resistance, whereas the acquired transposon carrying the *erm(X)* gene, which encodes an rRNA methyltransferase, is also involved in clindamycin, erythromycin and telithromycin resistance.

Cutibacterium acnes is present on the skin surface at low level and forms dominant resident bacteria of the sebaceous follicles. Acne vulgaris is not a result of a greater proliferation of all *C. acnes* strains, as patients with acne do not have more *C. acnes* in the follicles when compared with normal individuals. However, acne may be triggered by subset of *C. acnes* strains, the acne-associated phylotype IA1, probably aggravated by a hyperseborrheic environment.

A state of equilibrium exists within the skin microbiota and between different *C. acnes* subtypes, which is important in the regulation of skin homeostasis. Studies show that *S. epidermidis* is known to inhibit growth of *C. acnes* and inflammation induced by *C. acnes*.

An imbalance due to changes in physiological conditions between various skin community members is called as dysbiosis, this eventually leads to selection of more pathogenic *C. acnes* strains. A state of disrupted equilibrium within the microbiota of skin and intrinsic properties of *C. acnes* might activate innate immunity, resulting in inflammation.

Probiotics to bring equilibrium of skin microbiota, medications to work on biofilms, and/or acne-associated phylotypes are potential areas, which require to be explored.

Key Messages

- In the new taxonomic classification, P. acnes is renamed as Cutibacterium acnes (C. acnes), along with characterization of its phylogenetic cluster groups
- A state of disrupted equilibrium within the microbiota of skin and intrinsic properties of C. acnes might activate innate immunity, resulting in inflammation.

ARTICLE 127

The In Vitro Antimicrobial Evaluation of Commercial Essential Oils and their Combinations against Acne

Orchard A, van Vuuren SF, Viljoen AM, et al. The in vitro antimicrobial evaluation of commercially essential oils and their combinations against acne.
Int J Cosmet Sci. 2018;40(3):226-43.

Abstract

The various commercial essential oil combinations against the two pathogens, *Staphylococcus epidermidis* (ATCC 2223) and *Propionibacterium acnes* (ATCC 11827), which are responsible for acne, were assessed in this study. The oils, which exhibited significant antimicrobial activity among the essential oil combinations, were *Pogostemon patchouli* Benth. (patchouli), *Vetiveria zizanioides* (*V. zizanioides*), *Cinnamomum verum* (*C. verum*), and *Santalum* species (sandalwood). However, it was found that none of the essential oil combinations recommended in the aromatherapeutic literature of layman had any synergistic interactions.

COMMENT

Essential oils have been used in the treatment of acne and clinical studies have shown that they exhibit anti-acne effects. *Melaleuca alternifolia* Cheel (tea tree) and *Ocimum basilicum* L. (basil) have clinical evidence supporting their use in patients with acne. A review identified that though many oils have been used in the treatment of acne, only a few have been investigated in vitro. Essential oils are rarely used as single oil for topical treatment, and they are often used in combination with an intention to enhance their therapeutic efficacy. The essential oils are blended in a combination to enhance the therapeutic synergy.

The study was conducted to determine the efficacy of commercial essential oil combinations against the two pathogens, *Staphylococcus epidermidis* (ATCC 2223) and *Propionibacterium acnes* (ATCC 11827) responsible for acne, and also to assess the synergy and favorable oil combinations to be blended for better outcome.

The chemical compositions of most of the essential oils used in this study have been previously studied, and however, to identify the chemical profile of each essential oil, gas chromatography coupled to mass spectrometry (GC-MS) has been used. The essential oils used in the study were evaluated individually and in 1:1 combinations using the broth microdilution assay. The combinations, which had synergistic interactions, were investigated at various ratios and evaluated. The minimum inhibitory concentration (MIC) and the fractional inhibitory concentration index (ΣFIC) were calculated to assess the antimicrobial activity against both the pathogens that cause acne.

Cinnamomum zeylanicum Blume (cinnamon leaf) oil had higher activity against both the acne pathogens than the oil sample studied by Orchard, Sandasi probably due to the higher eugenol content, which is known to have antimicrobial activity. *C. verum* oil inhibited both the two acne pathogens strongly than either of the *C. zeylanicum* species, and mostly attributed to the presence of cinnamaldehyde, which appears to have an even stronger antimicrobial activity to that of eugenol. The antimicrobial activity of cinnamaldehyde contained in *C. burmannii* (cinnamon) against *S. epidermidis* was observed by Nuryastuti, van der Mei.

Cistus ladanifer L. 1 and 2, *Cymbopogon nardus* (L.) Rendle, and *Matricaria recutita* L. (German chamomile) displayed noteworthy antimicrobial activity against both the acne pathogens. *Mentha spicata* L.

(spearmint) demonstrated a stronger antimicrobial activity than that of *Mentha piperita* L. (peppermint) against *P. acnes* and moderate against *S. epidermidis*. *Pelargonium graveolens* L'Hér. had stronger antimicrobial activity than previously reported *Pelargonium odoratissimum* (Soland.) against both acne pathogens. The *Rosa damascena* Mill. samples exhibited equal noteworthy antimicrobial activity, and *Rosa centifolia* L. was earlier reported to inhibit *P. acnes* at an MIC of 0.03%. The two *Ocimum tenuiflorum* L. (holy basil) samples, in this study, inhibited *S. epidermidis* and *P. acnes* at noteworthy MIC most likely due to the higher eugenol content. *Origanum vulgare* L. (oregano) has potential anti-acne activity against the pathogens similar to the previous study against *S. epidermidis* strains. *Vetiveria* and *Santalum* species also exhibited good anti-acne potential.

About 167 of the 408 combinations, that were investigated, demonstrated noteworthy antimicrobial activity (MIC value ≤1.00 mg mL^{-1}).

Thirteen of the 19 essential oils, that were evaluated, inhibited *S. epidermidis* at a noteworthy concentration (MIC 1.00 mg mL^{-1} and less). *Vetiveria zizanioides* (vetiver), *Cinnamomum verum* J. Presl (cinnamon bark), and *Santalum austrocaledonicum* Vieill. (sandalwood) displayed the strongest activity with an MIC value of 0.25 mg mL^{-1}.

Eighteen out of 19 essential oils, that were evaluated, inhibited *Propionibacterium acnes* at a noteworthy concentration. The strongest antimicrobial activity against *P. acnes* with MIC values of 0.19 mg mL^{-1} and 0.13 mg mL^{-1} was exhibited by *Nardostachys jatamansi* (spikenard) and *C. verum*, respectively.

It was found that 13 synergistic interactions were observed against *S. epidermidis* and three synergistic combinations were observed against *P. acnes*. The oil that was most commonly involved in synergistic interactions against *S. epidermidis* was *Leptospermum scoparium* manuka. Synergistic interactions against both the pathogens were exhibited by *Cananga odorata* (Lam.) Hook.f. and Thomson (ylang–ylang). *Vetiveria zizanioides* Stapf (vetiver) with *Cinnamomum verum* J. Presl (cinnamon bark) exhibited the lowest MIC values of 0.19–0.25 mg mL^{-1} against both the pathogens. The oils, which exhibited significant antimicrobial activity toward the essential oil combinations, were *Pogostemon patchouli* (patchouli), *V. zizanioides*, *C. verum*, and *Santalum* species (sandalwood). However, it was found that none of the essential oil combinations recommended in the aroma-therapeutic literature of layman had any synergistic interactions, emphasizing the need for scientific validation of essential oil antimicrobial activity. There was no antagonism that was observed.

Key Messages

- *Pogostemon patchouli* Benth. (patchouli), *V. zizanioides*, *C. verum*, and *Santalum* species (sandalwood) exhibited significant antimicrobial activity toward the essential oil combinations
- The essential oil combinations recommended in the aroma-therapeutic literature of layman did not have any synergistic interactions.

ARTICLE 128

Seasonal Aggravation of Acne in Summers and the Effect of Temperature and Humidity in a Study in a Tropical Setting

Narang I, Sardana K, Bajpai R, et al. Seasonal aggravation of acne in summers and the effect of temperature and humidity in a study in a tropical setting.
J Cosmet Dermatol. 2018.

Abstract

Acne and acne flares have been influenced by high temperature and humidity in tropical areas. When patients with acne were questioned about aggravation, improvement, or no change in their acne with respect to the seasons, it was found that 47.95% of the patients had seasonal variation of acne. Summer aggravation was statistically significant. Temperature and humidity have a role in pathogenesis of acne and acne flare. In this study, it was found that the aggravation of acne was more in summer and rainy season.

COMMENT

Western literature is of the consensus that summer season and ultraviolet radiation benefit acne, although a study from India has found the opposite to be true. This was a cross-sectional study for a period of 1 year in a tertiary care hospital in Delhi conducted on acne patients seeking treatment for acne.

A total of 216 patients out of 387 were on irregular or inappropriate treatment or on topical or systemic treatment, which could aggravate acne. Thus, 171 patients with acne vulgaris (87 males and 84 females) between age group of 12 years and 32 years, with a minimal duration of acne for 1 year, were evaluated. Patients on monthly regular follow-up were evaluated for variation in acne severity, whereas in the rest, a question-based assessment was carried out. Patients had duration of acne ranging for 1-20 years. The comprehensive acne severity system was used to grade acne as almost clear, mild, moderate, severe, and very severe. Based on the climate in Delhi, the seasons were categorized as summer (April to June), rainy (July to September), winter (November to February), spring (March), and autumn (October). Aggravation, improvement or no change in acne with the seasons was recorded on questioning the patients. The improvement or worsening was graded as 1 (mild, <25%), 2 (moderate, 25-50%), 3 (severe, 50-75%), and 4 (very severe), and the specific season of this variation was noted. The mean temperature was 32.2°C, 31°C, and 15°C in summer, rainy, and winters, respectively. The mean humidity was 49.2%, 68.5%, and 79.7% in summer, rainy, and winters, respectively.

About 47.95% of the patients reported seasonal variation of acne, 40.4% of patients reported aggravation in summer of which 54.89% of patients had aggravation in summer only. The aggravation in winter and rainy season was seen in 6.42% and 1.16% of patients, respectively. The aggravation in summers and improvement in winter was seen in 4.09% of cases, whereas another 4.09% had aggravation both in summer and rainy. Patients did not show any seasonal change in spring and autumn. The aggravation in summer was statistically significant compared to rainy and winter, the comparison between rainy and winter was not statistically significant. This is consistent with studies from India, whereas western literature suggests that fewer patients seek treatment for acne in summer months. However, a study from Munich found that one-third of the patients (46 of 139) reported aggravation of acne in summer, another one-third had improvement in winter (44/139), and the other third did not notice any seasonal change (46/139).

Clinical observations suggest that acne worsens on exposure to tropical and subtropical climates. The effect of ambient temperature and humidity were assessed by ruling out the history of usage of comedogenic agents, treatment taken for acne, and medications used, which could have aggravated acne. A higher mean temperature in summer had a flare in acne, as sebum excretion rate is directly proportional to change in local temperature; 1°C change in temperature produced a change in the sebum excretion in the order of 10%. Another contributory factor for flare in summer could possibly be ultraviolet A (UVA) light from the observation that photochemotherapy (PUVA) treatment can cause perioral dermatitis and acneiform eruption. On exposure to UVA, squalene gets converted to squalene monohydroperoxide, and this appears to be responsible for comedogenicity. The surface lipid had less squalene when forehead temperature was decreased, whereas no variations in the other components of the surface lipid were observed. Lower lipid production in winter was observed in another study corresponding to the observation in the present study.

Tropical acne was seen in troops during the Second World War who were posted in the Far East, which was similar to ambient high humidity in Delhi. The poral occlusive effect of skin in humid environment and friction irritating the upper parts of pilosebaceous duct may also contribute to acne. The improvement in acne during summers seen in this study may not be true for all geographical locations. The flare in acne in tropical conditions may be an effect of variation in temperatures and high humidity. If a flare is anticipated then therapy can be regulated, and also the effect of change in the temperature and humidity on acne influences the results of the trials with both topical and systemic agents for treating acne.

Key Messages

- Temperature and humidity both have a role in the pathogenesis of acne and are responsible for acne flare
- In this study, aggravation of acne was more in summer and rainy seasons.

ARTICLE 129

Acne Prevalence in 9–14-year-old Patients Attending Pediatric Ambulatory Clinics in Italy

Napolitano M, Ruggiero G, Monfrecola G, et al. Acne prevalence in 9 to 14-year-old patients attending pediatric ambulatory clinics in Italy.
Int J Dermatol. 2018;57(11):1320-3.

Abstract

In the present-day scenario, a higher proportion of patients with younger onset of acne vulgaris are commonly seen than in the past. When a total of 683, 9–14-year-old, patients attending 32 different ambulatory clinics in Italy were analyzed, it was found that acne was present in 34.3% of the patients. About 88.5% of patients suffering from acne had mild disease state severity. Around 1.7% of patients had severe or very severe forms of acne.

COMMENT

Acne vulgaris is a chronic inflammatory disease of the pilosebaceous follicles affecting patients of all ages. Adolescents and adults, aged 12-24 years, are the most commonly affected with a prevalence of 70-80%. However, recent literature shows that younger age of onset is common, with an increasing earlier age of onset in childhood between 1 year and 8 years of age. Childhood acne is now considered as a normal variant of acne not requiring endocrinological evaluation as against the earlier belief.

Various factors, including hormones, body mass index (BMI), and diet, may contribute to the pathogenesis of acne. A prospective observational study was conducted for 12 months to evaluate acne in childhood/preadolescent age in 32 different pediatric ambulatory clinics and to investigate the prevalence, clinical features, risk factors, and treatments of acne in 9–14-year-old patients.

Out of 683 children, 49.2% were males and 50.8% being females, 11.05 ± 1.4 years was the mean age of the study population, 98.8% were Caucasian. About 33.1% of female subjects had attained menarche as against 11% of male patients had spermarche. History of acne was recorded in 10.4% of the patients, history of neonatal acne was found in 6.7%, infantile, and mid-childhood acne in 1.0% and 2.6%, respectively. At pediatric consultation, 34.3% of the patients had acne, which was similar to the one report in Korean children (36.2%) but higher when compared to a report from Taiwan (17.5%).

Acne prevalence increased with age, being lowest at 9 years (6%) and higher after 13 years (6%) of age, which is comparable to the prevalence of inflammatory acne in the age group of 7-9 years, reported from Taiwan (between 1.8% and 3.9%).

Although acne was more common in females and it did not approach statistical significance (59.4% females), even menarche was associated with childhood/preadolescent acne without reaching statistical significance (52.5%). Spermarche did not have any statistically significance in acne patients. In this study, 47.5% of girls and 73.6% of boys with acne did not present menarche or spermarche, respectively, showing that acne can frequently appear before puberty, which is similar to earlier report that higher number of comedones or inflammatory lesions before the onset of puberty is closely related to subsequent development of severe acne.

The face (98.7%) was the most common site of involvement, followed by the trunk (16.3%) and the neck (8.2%). Younger children had lesions on the cheeks and older children on the face, which reflect the natural course of acne as it starts with predominantly noninflammatory lesions, followed by an increase in inflammatory lesions, and it also has a wider distribution.

Mild or almost clear disease severity (GEA scale 1 or 2) was found in 88.5% of patients, suggesting that moderate to severe forms of the disease are very rare in preadolescent age. The severe or very severe forms (GEA scale 4 or 5) were found only in 1.7% of the cases. About one-fourth (21.4%) of the patients were on pharmacologic therapy for acne, and half (56.4%) of the patients were on dermocosmetic therapy prescribed by the pediatrician. A dermatological consultation was done by 25.9% of the patients, whereas pediatricians prescribed pharmacological acne therapy in 74.1% and dermocosmetic treatment in 91.3% of the cases.

Some studies report that approximately one-third of the children who had used some type of acne treatment based on a pharmacy visit, cosmetics, or self-medication instead of visiting a dermatologist or a pediatrician. This reflects inadequate treatment seeking behavior. The topical antibiotics were the most common prescribed treatment in acne patients (29.6%), followed by benzoyl peroxide (22.2%), topical retinoids with benzoyl peroxide (18.5%), azelaic acid (18.5%), and systemic antibiotics (14.8%), whereas dermocosmetic treatments consisted of specific soaps (96.6%), creams (39.8%), and moisturizers (31.8%).

An endocrine or metabolic evaluation may be needed, if there are signs of hyperandrogenism or sexual precocity. Tetracyclines should be avoided in children less than 8 years of age and isotretinoin is primarily used in adults above 12 years of age or older. The exceptions for isotretinoin include an infant or child with severe or recalcitrant, nodulocystic acne that is likely to develop scarring. The use of oral contraceptive and hormonal therapies for acne should be reserved for women who have been menstruating for at least 1 year. Although these patients have a mild disease, the possibility of worsening should be kept in mind and adequate treatment should be ensured. Early control of childhood acne helps to minimize the impact of the disease on the patient, as acne may persist over years.

Key Messages

- *Acne is not a rare disease in the preadolescent population*
- *Adequate treatment is needed in this group of patients to minimize the disease burden and avoid the possibility of worsening of acne.*

ARTICLE 130

Confocal Microscopy in Adult Women with Acne

Muguet Guenot L, Vourc'h Jourdain M, Saint-Jean M, et al. Confocal microscopy in adult women with acne.
Int J Dermatol. 2018;57(3):278-83.

Abstract

Reflectance confocal microscopy (RCM) was done to assess infundibulum morphology in adult women with acne. Apparently, healthy forehead skin of adult women with acne showed follicles with larger diameter, thicker, and hyperkeratinized follicle border, and more keratin plugs compared with the healthy skin of healthy adult women. The mandibular-affected skin showed follicles, which were significantly larger, thicker, more hyperkeratinized, with more keratin plugs and increased inflammation compared to apparently healthy forehead skin in a given patient.

COMMENT

Acne affects 41–54% of women above 25 years of age. Mixed facial acne involving several areas (89.8%) and acne localized to the mandible (11.2%) are the two types of adult acne. There are two types, continuous acne with an onset in adolescence that may include periods of remission, and in 20% of cases, adult-onset acne appearing between the age of 25 years and 40 years.

Follicular hyperkeratinization, sebum composition alteration, sebum hyperproduction, proliferation of *Propionibacterium acnes* (*P. acnes*), hormonal dysregulation, and chronic inflammation are the various etiologies resulting in acne. The microcomedo is considered the first histological lesion in acne and *P. acnes* could play a role by modulating keratinocyte differentiation and proliferation.

Reflectance confocal microscopy is a noninvasive tool allowing instantaneous visualization of skin structures at a cellular-level resolution. The study was done in adult women over 20 years of age divided into two groups. The severity of acne was determined by the Global Evaluation Acne (GEA) scale. Clinical count of comedones, papules, pustules, and nodules was done. Seborrhea was given a scoring of 0 for no seborrhea and 4 for severe. Women without history of acne were taken as control.

Two groups of 15 adult women with acne were included in an 18-months study. The first group consisted of 15 patients with diffuse acne lesions on face involving the forehead, cheeks, and chin. On a visually healthy skin of forehead, two 3 × 3 mm Vivacubes were obtained using VivaScope® 1500. The same was obtained from 6 adult women with no history of acne.

The second group had 15 patients with mandibular acne, who were their own control to compare the lesion-free forehead area and the involved mandibular area. Two 3 × 3 mm Vivacubes were obtained, one over the acne-free forehead region and the other over the mandibular area with acne. The same was obtained from 6 adult women with no history of acne.

The first group of 15 women with diffuse acne, when assessed on the healthy skin over the forehead, showed follicles with larger diameter, thicker (68%), and hyperkeratinized follicle border (65%), and more keratin plugs (44%) than healthy skin in healthy controls. Signs of inflammation were seen in 19.6% of follicles in patients with acne in group one compared to 9.2% in the controls.

Second group of 15 adult women with acne over mandibular zone showed follicles over the mandible, which were significantly larger, thicker (76%), more hyperkeratinized (72%), with more keratin plugs (47%) and increased inflammation (23%), compared with the healthy forehead skin in a given patient. The control group did not show any difference in the follicles on the forehead and the mandible except the keratin plugs were more on forehead.

Adult women with acne had higher hyperkeratinization over healthy forehead skin compared to healthy skin of adult women. Hyperkeratinization has an "onion-peel" like appearance on confocal microscope and plugs of keratin corresponds to microcomedo histologically. These reflect keratinization abnormalities of the follicle epithelium associated with an increased Ki-67 proliferative index and abnormal expression of keratin 6 and 16. The evaluation of the first group showed that the inflammatory signs were common around the follicle of the apparently healthy skin of adult patients with acne (19.6%), which were in accordance with the results found by Jeremy et al. Jeremy et al. showed the presence of CD3, CD4 T lymphocytes, and macrophages in the perifollicular area on the normal skin of patients with acne. An early infundibular inflammation along with the development of microcomedo is one of the initiating events of acne lesion formation in the "diffuse subtype" of adult and juvenile acne. Hence, treating both patient's normal skin and acne lesions is necessary.

Adult women with acne involving mandible were associated with early impairments of follicles developed specifically in the mandibular region compared with the forehead. The mandibular region not only had inflammatory lesions (deep cysts), but comedones and microcomedones (47%) were appreciable by confocal microscopy. Only about 0.2% of follicles had inflammation without hyperkeratinization in the mandibular area compared with 15.3% with both a thickened border with an onion-peel like appearance and a keratin plug associated with inflammation. With the above findings, it is evident that inflammatory signs seem closely related to hyperkeratinization. Isolated inflammation without hyperkeratinization was never observed. This in favor of the hypothesis that hyperkeratinization is the first cause for acne even in the mandibular inflammatory subtype of acne. Hence, the use of comedolytic should be ensured clinically.

Key Messages

- Microcomedo is essential for the development of acne lesions, hence, the importance of treating the entire skin surface with a topical treatment in adult acne
- Although clinically inflammatory lesions are more commonly seen in mandibular acne, higher number of follicular alterations stress the role of microcomedo and comedo in mandibular acne.

ARTICLE 131

Erythema-directed Digital Photography for the Enhanced Evaluation of Topical Treatments for Acne Vulgaris

Micali G, Dall'Oglio F, Tedeschi A, et al. Erythema-directed digital photography for the enhanced evaluation of topical treatments for acne vulgaris.
Skin Res Technol. 2018;24(3):440-4.

Abstract

Erythema-directed digital photography is a novel approach to evaluate the efficacy and tolerability of topical acne treatments. Three cases of acne in which standard clinical photography and erythema-directed digital photography (VISIA-CR™ system) were used to evaluate acne lesions and erythema, before and after up to 12 weeks of treatment with clindamycin 1%/tretinoin 0.025% (Clin-RA), have been reported. There was a clear improvement in background erythema and a reduction in acne lesions following treatment with Clin-RA.

COMMENT

Lesion counting and global disease assessments are used to evaluate acne and the impact of topical treatments. Clinical lesion counting can be subjective to individual assessors, only assesses what is visible to the naked eye, difficult to reliably identify minimal inflammatory lesions and to differentiate between papules and early pustules. The evaluation of local side effects such as erythema, which may occur in up to 70% of patients treated with topical retinoids, is usually missed in clinical assessments. Advanced digital photography techniques may be able to supplement simple clinical assessments.

Three 12-week pivotal clinical studies involving 4,550 patients have shown that clindamycin 1%/tretinoin 0.025% (Clin-RA) is well tolerated and effective at reducing inflammatory, noninflammatory, and total acne lesions compared with its monotherapy and vehicle components. In comparison with the monotherapy and car treatment groups, local side effects such as erythema, burning, scaling, stinging, and itching with Clin-RA were no higher than and moderate in intensity. The patented, aqueous gel formulation and the presence of both solubilized and crystalline tretinoin in Clin-RA lead to favorable tolerability profile. Crystalline retinoid is slowly released on the skin surface allowing sustained cutaneous penetration.

The three patients with mild-to-moderate facial acne vulgaris (AV) reported here were treated once-daily for 8-12 weeks with a topical gel containing Clin-RA. They were evaluated before and after treatment using standard clinical photography and the VISIA-CR™ system (Canfield Scientific Inc., Fairfield, NJ, USA). The erythema-directed imaging highlights areas of redness corresponding to increased vascular flare or inflammation.

Patient 1 was 18-year old with mild facial acne for 1 year and had been treated with benzoyl peroxide 5% gel for 4 months. Patient 2 was a 17-year-old male with moderate facial acne for 8 months and had received clindamycin 1%/benzoyl peroxide 5% for 2 months. Patient 3 was a 22-year-old female with untreated mild facial acne for 6 months. Patient 1 and 2 refused treatment due to irritation in addition patient 2 also had poor response. Patient 1, 2, and 3 showed improvement at 12, 8, and 8 weeks, respectively on comparison of the standard clinical photographs and erythema-directed digital images. Background erythema in patients 1 and 2 due to previous treatment had also improved.

In patient 3, comparison of the standard clinical photograph with the erythema-directed digital image shows that the latter allows a better visualization of the patient's noninflammatory lesions, closed comedones, appearing as white spots. Clinical and erythema-driven pictures of the patient 3 showed a marked improvement in both inflammatory and noninflammatory lesions after 8 weeks of therapy with Clin-RA. The cases presented here show that erythema-directed digital photography can enhance the evaluation of the effects of topical treatments on acne and allow more accurate assessment of patients' acne lesions compared with clinical assessment alone. Erythema-directed digital photography allows accurate assessment of both inflammatory and noninflammatory lesions, and erythema before and after treatment. Imaging allows clear differentiation of erythema related to active acne lesions and that resulting from previous treatments (background erythema).

The tolerability of treatment can be assessed easily by determining the changes in background erythema.

The VISIA-CR™ system used in this study has previously been used to accurately and reproducibly, autoclassify and count inflammatory and noninflammatory acne lesions. This avoids the tedious and subjective process of manual lesion counting. Patient 1 and 2 had irritation with previous treatment, which was evident as background erythema. However, both patients had a marked improvement in their acne, as well as an improvement in erythema after switching to Clin-RA. These instances confirm that Clin-RA is not an irritant and that patients are well tolerated owing to its distinctive structure and mixture of solubilized and crystalline tretinoin to slowly release the retinoid on the surface of the skin. Three pivotal studies of this fixed combination showed that Clin-RA was better tolerated than adapalene 0.1%/benzoyl peroxide 2.5% being associated with significantly less burning/stinging and itching ($p < 0.001$) as well as significantly lower transepidermal water loss, an objective measure of skin irritation. Another 3-week research showed that Clin-RA was better tolerated than 0.1% tretinoin microsphere gel, a retinoid deemed to be highly tolerable. Fixed combinations containing two antimicrobial agents are regarded as suboptimal as they lack a retinoid to target the microcomedone. The Global Alliance to Improve Outcomes in Acne group recommends fixed-dose combinations that combine a retinoid with an antimicrobial agent for most acne patients as they are associated with faster and more effective lesion clearance than monotherapies.

> **Key Messages**
> - Erythema-directed digital photography enhances the evaluation of the efficacy and tolerability of topical acne treatments
> - In this study, Clin-RA showed an improved efficacy and tolerability versus previous treatments with topical monotherapy (benzoyl peroxide 5%) or a topical fixed-dose combination (clindamycin 1%/benzoyl peroxide 5%).

ARTICLE 132

Acne Vulgaris: The Metabolic Syndrome of the Pilosebaceous Follicle

Melnik BC. Acne vulgaris: The metabolic syndrome of the pilosebaceous follicle.
Clin Dermatol. 2018;36(1):29-40.

Abstract

The prevalence rates of acne are higher in developed countries. No acne has been found in non-Westernized populations still living under Paleolithic dietary conditions. Western diet overstimulates mechanistic target of rapamycin complex 1 (mTORC1). Increased mTORC1 activity has been detected in lesional skin and sebaceous glands of patients with acne. Obesity, type 2 diabetes mellitus (T2DM), cancer, and neurodegenerative diseases exhibit increased mTORC1 signaling, which is a characteristic feature of insulin resistance. Acne vulgaris (AV) is a member of mTORC1-driven diseases of civilization.

COMMENT

In non-Westernized populations, living under Paleolithic dietary conditions and constraining hyperglycemic carbohydrates, milk, and dairy products, no acne has been found. High intake of sugar and other hyperglycemic carbohydrates, milk, and other dairy products are a characteristic of a Neolithic western diet. The above diet increases the insulin, insulin-like growth factor 1 (IGF-1), and mechanistic target of rapamycin complex 1 (mTORC1) signaling, which have been implicated as playing a key role in pathogenesis. Insulin/IGF-1 signaling growth, and anabolism are promoted by the branched-chain essential amino acids (BCAAs), which activate the growth factor and nutrient-sensitive kinase mTORC1. A Western diet also includes excessive amounts of essential BCAAs, which contribute to overstimulation of mTORC1 signaling.

Hyperglycemic carbohydrates induce postprandial rise of serum insulin levels and insulin signals activating mTORC. Milk transfers microRNAs that are transported via exosomes, which target and inhibit the expression of DNA methyltransferase 1 (DNMT1) and DNMT3B. DNMT inhibition increases the expression of nuclear factor erythroid 2-related factor, which promotes the expression of mTOR. mTOR is the core component of the mTORC1 and mTORC2 complexes.

Palmitic acid is abundant in dietary fat and milk lipids. Palmitic acid activates mTORC1 at the lysosomal membrane, the same location where BCAAs activate mTORC1. In the skin of patients with acne, there is enhanced expression of mTOR and activated S6K1. Increased signaling of mTORC1 activates kinase S6K1, which creates insulin resistance through phosphorylation of IRS-1. Adiponectin improves insulin sensitivity and activates AMP kinase, leading to inhibition of mTORC1. Low expression of adiponectin sebocytes of patients with acne enhances mTORC1 signaling and further insulin resistance.

Testosterone and dihydrotestosterone have a role in sebaceous lipogenesis, sebaceous gland hypertrophy, and acne vulgaris. Androgen receptor (AR) signaling increases the activity of mTORC2, which activates the kinase AKT, similar to insulin and IGF-1. AR negatively regulates the expression of DEP domain-containing mTOR-interacting protein (DEPTOR), a natural inhibitor of mTORC1 and mTORC2.

The mTORC1 plays an important role for the translation of the key transcription factor of sebaceous lipogenesis sterol regulatory element-binding protein 1 (SREBP1). SREBP1 and AR, the transcription factors, are both repressed in the nucleus by the metabolic transcription factor FoxO1. Nuclear FoxO1 activity is inhibited by enhanced insulin/IGF-1 signals in human sebocytes and sebaceous glands in patients with acne. There is not only a quantitative change of sebum (hyperseborrhea) but also qualitative modifications of sebum (dysseborrhea) with an increase of monounsaturated fatty acids promote acne pathogenesis.

Most fatty acids are covalently bound in triacylglycerol in ordinary sebum. The quantities of complete free fatty acids produced in acne patients are more than 50% greater than those of age-matched controls without acne. Triacylglycerol lipase releases the free fatty acids, which is a virulence factor of *Propionibacterium acnes* that is upregulated in *P. acnes* biofilm.

Free oleic acid has been found to enhance calcium influx into epidermal keratinocytes, increase keratinocyte proliferation, and induce abnormal keratinization and barrier function associated with increased release of interleukin (IL)-1α, which play a crucial role in comedogenesis. Oleic acid, squalene, and their peroxides cause relatively big comedones in the follicular infundibulum associated with marked epithelial hyperplasia and hyperkeratosis. Palmitic acid-mediated TLR2 activation increases the expression of NLRP3 and induces inflammasome-mediated IL-1β production, IL-1β expression is upregulated in sebaceous glands of acne lesions.

Fatty acid metabolism is involved in T-helper 17 (Th17) cell differentiation. Acetyl-CoA carboxylase 1 (ACC1), which is the rate-limiting enzyme of sebaceous de novo fatty acid synthesis, has been found to favor Th17 cell development over regulatory T cells in mice. SREBP1, which is an mTORC1-dependent lipogenic transcription factor, induces expression of ACC1. Sebum-derived fatty acids, especially free oleic acid, promote a Th17-regulated inflammatory microenvironment of the sebaceous follicle observed in acne vulgaris.

The most effective treatment for acne, isotretinoin, does not attenuate sebocyte metabolic activity but causes sebocyte-induced apoptosis. The activity of mTOR is reduced by topical application of the ACC inhibitor olumacostat glasaretil (OG), eicosapentaenoic acid (EPA), and docosahexaenoic acid (DHA). Polyphenols, derived from plants such as epigallocatechin-3-gallate in green tea and resveratrol in grapes and berries, also inhibit mTORC1. The substitution of vitamin D in acne leads to attenuation of mTORC1 signaling, which may reduce sebum production and increase the expression of the antimicrobial peptide cathelicidin, which is able to kill *P. acnes*.

To conclude, there is a need for medications that attenuate mTORC1/SREBP1-mediated sebum production by regulation of mTORC1- and FoxO1-dependent signaling pathways.

Key Messages
- Acne vulgaris has been identified as a member of the family of mTORC1-driven metabolic diseases, such as obesity, type 2 diabetes mellitus, and cancer, and is a disease of Western civilization
- A western diet, especially hyperglycemic load and milk consumption, increases mTORC1/SREBP1 signaling, and IGF-1–mediated mTORC1 activation during puberty, which eventually leads to acne vulgaris.

ARTICLE 133

Circular RNA Expression Profile Analysis of Severe Acne by RNA-Seq and Bioinformatics

Liang J, Wu X, Sun S, et al. Circular RNA expression profile analysis of severe acne by RNA-Seq and bioinformatics. *J Eur Acad Dermatol Venereol.* 2018;32(11):1986-92.

Abstract
Acne is a chronic inflammatory disease of pilosebaceous units. In recent past, circular RNAs (circRNAs) have been known to play a role in many biological processes and human diseases by regulating gene expression through circRNA-miRNA-mRNA networks. This study was done to investigate circRNA expression profile in severe acne and the circRNAs were differentially expressed in severe acne. The circRNAs could be used as a potential biomarker for developing newer drugs to treat acne.

COMMENT

Acne, a chronic skin disease, characterized by inflammatory, noninflammatory lesions, seborrhea, and/or various degrees of scarring, has multifactorial etiology and pathogenesis. In recent past, circular RNAs (circRNAs) have been known to play a role in many biological processes and human diseases by regulating gene expression through circRNA-miRNA-mRNA networks. Since, the circRNAs expression in patients with acne is still unknown, this study was done to investigate circRNA expression profile in severe acne.

A total of 7 subjects with clinical diagnosis of severe acne (grade IV) confirmed by two dermatologists were included in the study. A paired lesional and adjacent nonlesional skin located about 2 cm from the affected area was taken from each subject. The samples from three males with a mean age of 22.3 years were subjected to RNA-seq analysis. The samples collected from 4 males with a mean age of 21.0 years were analyzed by polymerase chain reaction (PCR), Sanger sequencing, and qRT-PCR.

Three paired lesion skin and adjacent nonlesional skin in severe acne patients were assessed and expression profile of circRNAs was detected by high-throughput RNA sequencing technology and bioinformatics analysis. The validation of candidate circRNAs was done by PCR, Sanger sequencing, and qRT-PCR, and the circRNA-miRNA-mRNA interaction networks were predicted.

There were 271 upregulated and 267 downregulated circRNAs, a total of 538 circRNAs, which were differentially expressed in lesional skin compared with adjacent nonlesional skin in severe acne. Gene Ontology and KEGG pathway enrichment analyses were done, which showed that the aberrantly expressed circRNAs were primarily involved in inflammatory, metabolism, and immune responses. When PCR, Sanger sequencing, and qRT-PCR were done, 5 candidate circRNAs (circRNA_0084927, circRNA_0001073, circRNA_0005941, circRNA_0086376, and circRNA_0018168) were validated to have significant decrease in severe acne, similar to the results from RNA-Seq data analysis. These 5 circRNAs, that were identified, were predicted to interact with 213 circRNAs. The identified circRNAs also regulated target gene expression.

The circRNAs were differentially expressed in severe acne and could be used as a potential biomarker for developing newer drugs to treat acne.

Key Messages

- The circRNAs were differentially expressed in severe acne
- The circRNAs could be used as a potential biomarker for developing newer drugs to treat acne.

ARTICLE 134

Taxonomy and Phylogeny of *Cutibacterium* (formerly *Propionibacterium*) *acnes* in Inflammatory Skin Diseases

Corvec S, Dagnelie MA, Khammari A, et al. Taxonomy and phylogeny of *Cutibacterium* (formerly *Propionibacterium*) *acnes* in inflammatory skin diseases.
Ann Dermatol Venereol. 2019;146(1):26-30.

Abstract

Propionibacterium acnes is termed as *Cutibacterium acnes* after undergoing various term changes since its discovery. *Cutibacterium* includes five species within the cutaneous ecosystem. Finer distinction between species and subspecies is done with modern microbiological techniques, which also enables the identification of separate subtypes within the population of *Cutibacterium acnes*. Phylogeny and molecular typing techniques thus provide a better understanding of the subtypes involved in acne.

COMMENT

Propionibacterium acnes is one of the predominant bacteria found within the pilosebaceous follicles and their orifices. It forms part of the cutaneous microbiota. Propionic acid from lactose is fermented under anaerobic conditions to give an acidic cutaneous pH that hampers the implantation of pathogenic bacteria such as *Staphylococcus aureus* and *Streptococcus pyogenes*. All the earlier types of cutaneous *Propionibacterium* are now subsumed under a new bacterial genus named *Cutibacterium*. Within the population of *C. acnes* and its subtypes, which were initially determined by partial sequencing of the genes *recA* and *tly*, genomic techniques have enabled the identification of six phylogenetic groups—IA1, IA2, IB, IC, II and III. The development of acne is not correlated with an increase in the relative abundance of *C. acnes* in pilosebaceous follicles. It is more of an imbalance of the bacterial flora within the same subgroups of *C. acnes*, with loss of diversity of the subgroups and over-representation of a single phylotype, particularly phylotype IA1. The host plays an important role in terms of the composition of individual sebum, microbiota, and activation levels of innate immunity. Through their interaction with toll-like receptors (TLR), particularly TLR2 and TLR4, strains of *C. acnes* stimulate innate immunity. Interactions within the microbiota have recently been found to have a major role in the physiopathology of this chronic inflammatory skin disease with a new key factor—*Staphylococcus epidermidis*. *Staphylococcus epidermidis* acts on homeostasis of the cutaneous microbiota by interacting with the different phylogenetic groups of *C. acnes*. Thus, microbial balance of the skin is partly related to the action of each species bacteriocins active against other species. Simple cases of folliculitis of the scalp have shown clones of *C. acnes* similar to those found in acne and, in particular, those belonging to phylotype IA1 and to clonal complex CC18, while *C. namnetense* tended to be associated rather with Quinquaud's folliculitis decalvans. *S. aureus* is more commonly demonstrated in folliculitis keloidalis of the neck (acne keloidalis nuchae), and probably forms the source of the chronic suppuration associated with the pathogenic potency of this bacteria, which is also involved in atopic dermatitis. *C. acnes* phylotype III belonging to clonal complex CC43 has been shown to be present in progressive macular hypomelanosis (PMH). A therapeutic regimen effective against PMH (lymecycline and benzoyl peroxide) is associated with a change in the composition of the *C. acnes* population consisting of a considerable reduction in the proportion of *C. acnes* type III. Thus, restoration of balance in the distribution of phylotypes of *C. acnes* results in clinical improvement. These findings suggest the possibility of new therapeutic approaches using pre- or probiotics in cutaneous diseases involving such imbalance in bacterial communities of *C. acnes*.

Key Messages
- All the former types of cutaneous Propionibacterium are now subsumed under a new bacterial genus named Cutibacterium
- New therapeutic approaches using pre- or probiotics in cutaneous diseases restoring balance in the distribution of phylotypes of C. acnes result in clinical improvement.

ARTICLE 135

Transforming Acne Care by Pediatricians: An Interventional Cohort Study

Borok J, Udkoff J, Vaida F, et al. Transforming acne care by pediatricians: An interventional cohort study. *J Am Acad Dermatol.* 2018;79(5):966-8.

Abstract
Acne is a common disorder in adolescents and is treated by dermatologists and pediatricians. There is a major practice gap in the prescriptions of dermatologists and pediatricians. Pediatricians prescribe more of topical antibiotics as compared to dermatologists whose topical prescriptions are predominantly for retinoid. An intervention study was planned, where an educational program and electronic medical record (EMR) ordering tool was provided to pediatricians to improve the acne care.

COMMENT

Acne is predominantly a disorder of adolescence. Many pediatricians treat acne; however, there is a vast difference in prescription patterns of pediatricians and dermatologists. To provide pediatricians with an opportunity to treat acne effectively, an interventional cohort study was designed. A guideline-based education program was provided to pediatricians along with electronic medical record (EMR) tool, which provided medication recommendation based on the severity of acne. Survey was done to assess physician attitude and work burden on them.

After this intervention, the EMR tool was ordered 546 times, and a significant decrease in referrals to dermatologists for acne was noted. The prescription for retinoids was significantly higher than topical clindamycin. Acne causes severe psychological morbidity and scarring, a great amount of stress. If acne is treated effectively, the risk of scarring decreases significantly. Training pediatricians helps them to treat acne effectively and provide better acne care for patients. The referral to dermatologists also reduces.

Key Message

- Training pediatricians to treat acne improves the acne care given to patients at primary healthcare level.

INDEX

A

Acanthosis nigricans 177
Acetyl-CoA carboxylase-1 201
Acne 112, 162
  adolescents with 111
  aggravation 129
  agminata 19
  and dysmenorrhea, treatment of 54-56
  and nutrition 127
  associated phylotypes 189
  care by pediatricians 205
  clinical efficacy 49
  common disorder of adolescence 11
  conglobata of buttocks 17
  development of 13
  diagnostic criteria for 126
  etiopathogenesis of 5
  excoriee 41
  exposome factors 138
    climatic conditions 139
    mechanical factors 139
    medications 138
    nutrition 138
    occupational factors 138
    pollutants 139
  female patients with 42
  flares 192
  hypertrophic scar formation 156
  impact of 99
  in adult female diagnosis of 59
  in Lomé, Togo 102
  inflammatory process of 126
  keloidalis nuchae 205
  late-onset 92, 113
  light therapies for 46
  like phenotypes 150, 152
  management of 7, 48, 128
  mediated cytokine production 118
  medications 103, 104
  microbiome 149
  mild-to-moderate 9
  moderate 10, 71
  new concepts 146
  on back 158
  pathogenesis of 155, 193
  pipeline 147
  potential treatment of 48
  prevalence 194
  recurrence 92
  relapses quality of life 112
  relapsing 92
  related post-inflammatory hyperpigmentation, survey of 41
  scars 43, 49, 65, 79, 147
    management of 50, 82
    prevention of 132
    procedures 74
    treatment 86, 87
  severe, management of 56
  severity 105, 113, 123, 150
  skin, lesion-free 123
  specific quality of life 89
  susceptibility to 167
  symptoms 186
  therapy 85
  treatment of 22, 38
  vulgaris 1, 2, 15, 24, 40, 44, 57, 62, 63, 83, 84, 90, 92, 96, 109, 111, 113, 152, 171, 174, 176, 180, 183, 187, 200
    active 135
    burden of 165
    cognitive functions in adolescent 14
    evaluation of 198
    in Chinese population 173
    management technique for 24
    mild-to-moderate 69, 136
    moderate-to-severe 2, 3, 20, 83, 88, 163
    monotherapy in patients 7
    pathogenesis of 163, 178
    prevalence of 164, 165, 180
    severe, prognostic marker for 175
    severity 121
    stratum corneum of 11
    treatment of 10, 39, 75, 94, 96, 143, 198
  worsening of 195
Acneiform eruptions 18
Acrochordons 177
Actinobacteria 163, 164
Acylceramides 185, 187
Adapalene 43, 49, 50, 68, 96
  combination regimens of 9, 39, 96
  efficacy and safety of 9
  fixed combination 40
  gel group 73
  gel plus oral doxycycline 72
Adiponectin 201
Adipose tissue
  and function 176
  subcutaneous 176
Adrenal androgen inhibitors 93
Adult acne, female type of 91
Adult female acne 92
Adult-onset acne
  impact 29
  management challenges 29
  prevalence 29
Air pollutants 139
Allobaculum 163, 164
Aloe vera 38, 39
Alopecia, forms of 178

American Type Culture
    Collection 115
Aminolevulinic acid 69
    photodynamic therapy 72
    using 72
Aminomethylcycline 144
Ammonia-oxidizing bacteria
    102
Anabolic steroids trigger acne
    138
Androgen 145
    receptor signaling 201
Androgenetic alopecia 13, 177
    in male 13
Androgens synthesis of 126
Anorexia nervosa 128
Anti-acne isoprenylcysteine 169
Anti-acne therapy, development
    of 163
Antibacterial
    activity 169
    and anti-inflammatory
        activities 85, 153
Antibiotic tetracycline-class 147
Anticomedogenic 4
Anti-inflammatory
    action in vitro 160
    activity of 118, 159
    effects 159
    properties 143
        direct or indirect 86
    skin disease 154
Antimicrobial
    peptides 101
    resistance 169
    treatment 91
Antioxidative 4
Anti-tumor necrosis factor 18
Anxiety disorder, generalized
    112
Apigenin 91
    exhibited anti-inflammatory
        activity 91
Apoptosis marker 183, 185
Aromatherapy 58
Ascorbic acid 145
Atrophic acne scars 43, 64
    prevention 49
    reduction of 49
    severity of 181

treatment of 43, 78
volume of 182
Atrophic facial acne scars 25, 26
Attention deficit hyperactivity
    disorder 114
Autoimmune diseases 175
Autologous healthy hair follicles
    183
Automated chemiluminescent
    microparticle immunoassay
    124
Azelaic acid 4, 5, 30, 60
    efficacy and safety of 4

B

Bacillus subtilis 117
Bacteria
    colonization of 142
    host interactions 151
Bacterial
    resistance 132
        mechanisms of 132
    species 15
    toxins, group of 174
    concentration, minimum 169
Bacterium's nitrogen cycle 102
Bacteroidetes 164
Bacteroidiain 153
Barker-Gordon formula 71
Barriers to primary adherence
    103
Behcet's and psoriasis 153
Benzoyl peroxide 1, 9, 30, 35, 39,
    40, 47, 49, 50, 60, 68, 85, 93,
    96, 108, 169, 200, 205
    influence of 34
Bifidobacterium 67, 163, 164
Bisabolol isolated 91
Blood flow, assessments 123
Blood glucose, levels of 145
Blunt cannula
    procedure, using 87
    subcision 86, 87
Body dissatisfaction in
    adolescents 107
Body dysmorphic disorder 97,
    98
Body mass index 147, 180, 194
Boost procollagen fibroblast 147
Box scars 26

Branched-chain essential amino
    acids 200
Brassica oleracea var 90
Bulimia nervosa 112, 128
Butyricicoccus 163, 164

C

Candidiasis 144
Cannabis 139
Carboxytherapy 65
Cardiff acne disability index
    scores 77, 103
Cassia fistula 51
Cell culture 90
Cell surface hydrolase 188
Cell wall sugar analysis 101
Ceramide 121
    changes 185
    lower levels of 186
    species 186
Chamaecyparis obtusa 58
Cheilitis 45
Chemical peels 22, 53
    medium-depth 24
Chemical reconstruction of skin
    scars technique 74
Chlormadinone acetate 54, 55,
    138
Christie-Atkins-Munch-Petersen
    factor 148, 149
Cicatricial alopecia, primary 178
Cinnamomum verum 190, 191
Cinnamomum zeylanicum 190
CircRNA-miRNA-mRNA
    networks 202
Cistus ladanifer 190
Clindamycin 86, 137, 198, 200
Clindamycin benzoyl peroxide
    86
Clindamycin phosphate 1, 96
Clindamycin resistant 131
Clindamycin, treated group 137
Clostridia 153
Clostridiales 153
CO_2 laser 83
Coenzyme A desaturase-1 178
Coincubated undifferentiated
    human leukemia-derived
    monocytes 119
Coleman's combination 71

Collateral damage like dysbiosis 149
Colony forming unit 131
Comedogenic ingredients 138
Comedonal acne vulgaris, management of 85
Comedones, average number of 53
Comprehensive Acne Severity Scale 75
Confocal microscopy 161, 196
 in vivo reflectance 121
 reflectance 196
Copaiba oil 58
Copper-chelating agent 23
Coprobacillus 163, 164
Creatine kinase 146, 147
Crystalline precipitate 54
Cutaneous diseases 205
Cutaneous, types of 205
Cutibacterium 68, 101, 118, 131, 149, 169, 204
Cutibacterium acnes 4, 34, 130, 131, 143, 150, 187, 189, 204
 characterization of 130
 concentrations of 34
 growth of 3
 level of 36
 population of 204
Cutibacterium gen 188
Cutibacterium newly reclassified 118
Cutibacterium species 101
Cyproterone acetate 138

D

Dairy products 127
Damage-associated molecular pattern molecules 174
Danazol and dantrolene 18
Dapsone 7, 119
Dapsone gel
 tolerability of topical 10
 topical 19
Deeper epidermal 122
Dehydroepiandrosterone 29
Depression
 incidence of 22
 risk of 12, 14

Depressive disorder, major 12, 112
Depressive symptoms 107
Dermal matrix macromolecules 44
Dermal periphery 178
Dermal tissues 54
Dermatitis 18
Dermatological diseases, treatment of 37
Dermatologists, prescriptions of 205
Dermatology life quality index 108, 180
Dermis, removal of 179
Desquamation index 52
Diabetes mellitus, type 2 174, 176, 200
 insulin resistance with 175
Diaphoresis 18
Diatomaceous earth 62
Dienogest 138
Digital photography techniques, advanced 198
Dihydrotestosterone 29, 201
Diode laser 81, 95
 high-energy stamp-only regimen 80
Distinctive follicle infundibulum 122
Diversity, loss of 159
Docosahexaenoic acid 202
Doxycycline 9, 57, 68, 73, 143
 antipruritic efficacies of 75
 attenuates 76
Drospirenone 54, 55, 138
Dynamic cooling device 80, 81
Dysmenorrhea 55
Dysregulate epidermal differentiation 150, 152

E

Eating disorders 128
Échelle d'Evaluation Clinique des Cicatrices d'Acné scores 79
Échelle de Cotation des lésions d'acné score 103
Eicosapentaenoic acid 202
Electronic medical record 205

Emotional stress, periods of 110
Enzyme stearoyl-coenzyme A desaturase-1 68
Enzyme-linked immunosorbent assay 115, 176
 method 119
 technique 20
Epidermal
 barrier function, reduced 185
 ceramides 185
 growth factor 18, 65
 inflammation 123
 necrolysis 18
 opening 122
Epidermis 26, 78, 122, 134
Epigallocatechin-3-gallate 51, 202
Epithelial membrane antigen 179
EryR strains 131
Erythema 199
 directed digital photography 198, 200
Erythema index 52
Erythema multiforme 18
Erythroderma 18
Erythromycin 38, 75
Escherichia coli 90
Essential oils 59, 91, 138, 190
Estradiol 31
Ethinyl estradiol 55
 content of 55
 treated 108
Euphorbia supina 153, 154
European Academy of Dermatology and Venereology Task Forces 107
Evaluator's global severity score 88
Extracellular vesicles 151

F

Facial acne
 mild-to-moderate 85
 moderate 49
 severe 49
 vulgaris, treatment of 4
Facial adverse drug reactions 97
Facial idiopathic granulomas 19

Facial postinflammatory
    hyperpigmentation 106
    treatment of 106
Faster killing kinetics 160
Fatty acids 129, 159
    metabolism 201
    short-chain 188
Fatty acyls 120
Fecal samples 164
Feeling, uselessness of 107
Fermentation profiling 101
Fibrogenetic markers 156
Fibrosis of skin 157
Firmicutes 153, 164
Fistulas 165
Fitzpatrick skin, types of 1, 10,
    23, 82
Flavonoids 91
Follicle triggers inflammation
    101
Follicular hyperkeratinization
    171, 196
Follicular keratinocyte
    hyperproliferation 183
Follicular microbiome 154
Folliculitis, cases of 205
Forehead strips samplings 131
Fractional
    ablative carbon dioxide 65
    carbon dioxide laser 64
    microneedling radiofrequency
        78, 80, 95
Fragment length polymorphism
    171
Free fatty acids 121, 129
Free insulin like growth factor
    145, 176
Free oleic acid 202
Fructooligosaccharides 66
Fructooligosaccharides,
    supplementation with 66

G

Galactooligosaccharides 66
Galectin-7 11
Gamma-glutamyltransferase
    147
Gastrointestinal dysfunction 15
Gastrointestinal gram-negative
    bacteria 147

Gender dysphoria, symptoms
    of 31
Gender-specific triggers 92
Gene
    analysis, used for 90
    expression profile 133, 134
    ontology analysis 101
    polymorphisms, role of 166
Genetic
    factors 168
    susceptibility 142
Genome 142
Genomic techniques, advanced
    188
Genotyping of 174
Ginkgo biloba 51
Global acne grading scale, using
    135
Global acne grading system 33,
    77, 124, 140
    using 168
Global acne severity scale 112
Global evaluation acne scale 196
Global evaluation acne score
    150
Glycemic 66
Glycerolipids 121
Glycerophospholipids, levels
    of 120
Glycolic acid 74, 95
Glycyrrhiza inflata 162
    root of 162
Goodman and Baron's
    qualitative and quantitative
    global 82
Graft copolymer 37
Gram-positive bacterium 159
Granulocyte colony-stimulating
    factor 18
Gut microbiome
    analysis of 15
    components 15
Gut microbiota 163, 164
    alterations 163
Gut-brain-skin axis 102

H

Hair follicle 184
    content 123
Halogens 138

Hamilton anxiety rating scale
    110
Hamilton depression rating scale
    109, 110
Hamster sebocytes 178
Health improvement network
    database 12
Health-related quality of life 99,
    107
Healthy skin 187
Heat-killed *C. acnes* 102
Hepatotoxicity, concerns of 21
Herpes simplex flare-up 74
Hidradenitis suppurativa 164,
    165, 178, 180
High-glycemic diets 145
Hippophae rhamnoides 51
Hirsutism 43, 177
Homeostasis model assessment
    of insulin resistance index
    176
Hormonal antiandrogen
    acne, treatment 42
    therapy, use of 42
Hormonal treatment 2, 330
Hospital anxiety depression
    scale 77
Human-dependent pollutants
    139
Human epidermal keratinocytes
    150
Human immunodeficiency virus
    infection 175
Human intestine hosts 15
Human microbiome 143
Human sebaceous glands 134
Hurley score 180
Hydroalcoholic extract 91
Hyperandrogenemia 176
Hyperglycemic carbohydrates
    201
Hyperglycemic food 127
Hyperinsulinemia 176
    acute 66
    causes 176
    chronic 66
Hyperkeratinization 151
Hyperkeratotic follicular borders
    123
Hyper-reflective border 123

Hypertrophic scars
  immature 157
  pathogenesis of 156
Hypopigmentation 74
Hypotheses 127, 129

I

Ice-pick scars 182
IL-6 gene promoter
    polymorphism 139-141
Immune response mediator 166
Immune responses with plasma
    cells 132
Immune-mediated inflammatory
    skin conditions 18
Immunohistochemistry staining
    157
Immunosuppressants 138
Immunosuppressive drugs 164
Industrial pollutants 139
Infection and immunity 173
Inflammation 122
  in acne 159
  resulting in 189
Inflammatory acne
  average reduction of 137
  important in 163
Inflammatory cells
  density of 123
  using density of 123
Inflammatory cytokines 116
  IL-8 150
  secretion 129
  secretion of 152
Inflammatory disease
  action in 17
  chronic 83, 152, 194
Inflammatory disorder, chronic
    35
Inflammatory, expression of 156
Inflammatory lesions 88, 197
  reductions in 84
Inflammatory reaction 52
Inflammatory skin diseases 153
Infundibular border 123
Infundibular diameter 122, 123
Infundibular hyperkeratinization
    183
Inhibitory concentration,
    minimum 159, 169, 190

Innate immune system
  activating 174
  relies 174
Innate immunity 159
  activate 189
Insulin growth factor-1 138
Insulin-like growth factor-1 29,
    66
Intense inflammatory cytokine
    production 151
Intercellular cell adhesion
    molecule-1 115
Interferon-beta 18
Interleukin-1 beta 168
Interleukin-6 gene promoter
    polymorphism 139
International Classification of
    Diseases 114
Intestinal flora 143, 144
Intracellular lipids, levels of 130
Intraclass correlation 182
Investigator's
  global assessment 84, 172, 173
  static global assessment 97
Irisin 176
Isoniazid 138
Isotretinoin 9, 14, 21, 27, 33, 45,
    68, 78, 108, 124, 149
  for acne 56
  side effect of 14, 45
  therapy 16
Itch intensity 76

J

Jessner's solution, modified 71

K

Kaempferol 91
Keloidalis of neck 205
Keloids 74
Keratin 7 179
  plugs 197
Keratinocyte
  and cellular responses 151
  and sebocytes 124
  development 184
  hyperproliferation 128
  proliferation 183, 184
Keratotic content 123
Ketogenic diet 145

Kojic acid 23
Korean Acne Grading System 52
Koreans' acne skin 52

L

Lachnospiraceae 153
Lactic acid 23
Lactobacilli 67
Lactobacillus 58, 163, 164
Lactobacillus species 36
Laser and light therapies 147
Leveraging polymerized
    emulsion technology 88
Lichen planopilaris 178
Licochalcone 162
Life satisfaction 111
LifeViz captures 183
Light-based therapies 146
Lipid content 129
Lipid metabolic parameters 66
Lipocalin 11
Liquid chromatography-mass
    spectrometry 154
Lithium 138
Liver transaminases 147
Luciferase reporter, dual 174
Luteinizing hormone, levels of
    31
Lymecycline 205
Lymphocyte ratio 181

M

Macular hypomelanosis,
    progressive 205
Malassezia 101
Mandelic acid 23
Mandibular
  acne 197
  area 196
  line 30
Mangosteen, clinical efficacy
    of 136
Mangostin nanoparticle loaded
    gel 137
Mannitol 51
Masculinizing hormonal
  therapy 31
  side effect of 31
Matricaria chamomilla 90
Mean blood flow 123

Mechanical resurfacing techniques 147
Mediterranean diet 145
Melaleuca alternifolia 190
Mental health burden 113
Metabolic, evaluation of 195
Metabolic syndrome 176, 200
Metagenomic next-generation sequencing 150
Methacrylated hyaluronic acid 62
Methyl-ester methyl-aminolevulinate 46
Mice ears 159
Microbiome in preadolescent acne 34
Microcomedo 197
Microcomedones 64, 123, 197
Microneedle fractional radiofrequency 25, 26
Micro-organism index 52
Micro-plasma radiofrequency, using 78
Microscopic documentation 161
Microshort pulse mode 82
Microstructure skin analysis, used for 182
Milk
  consumption 68, 125
  products 126
Minocycline 57, 144, 147
Mitochondrial reactive oxygen species 162
Mitogenic growth factors 65
Mitosis 183
Monheit's combination 71
Myeloid cells 151
Myrtacine cream 130, 132
Myrtle essential oil, effects of 52

N

Nardostachys jatamansi 191
Natal female genitalia 22
Necrolytic acral erythema 18
Neolithic western diet 200
Neurodegenerative diseases 200
Neuropsychological test battery 14
Neutralizing antibodies 151
  using 152

Neutrophil gelatinase-associated lipocalin
  level of 11
  role of 11
Newcastle-Ottawa scale, using 126
Nicotinamide 36
  application of 37
  extrudates 36
Nitric oxide-releasing particles 68
Nitrosomonas eutropha 102
NLRP3
  gene 173
  inflammasomes 175
Nodule formation 182
Nokor needle subcision 86, 87
Nonadherence 16
Noninflammatory lesions 96, 199
Non-lesional skin, biopsies of 133
Nonpharmacological therapies, safety of 94
Non-scar-prone 133
Norethindrone acetate 108
Norgestimate 138
Novel tretinoin 2, 88
Nucleic acid leakage, measurement 160
Nucleocytoplasmic distribution 27
Nutrient-sensitive kinase 200

O

Okor needle subcision 86
Optical coherence tomography 121, 122
Oral contraceptives 55
Oral isotretinoin 146
Oxidative stress 46

P

Palmitic acid 129, 201
Papillary dermis 122
Papules 122
Pathogen-associated molecular pattern molecules 174
Patient satisfaction score 88
Pediatric ambulatory clinics 194

Pelargonium graveolens 191
Pelargonium odoratissimum 191
Persistent acne 92, 113
Phosphate buffered saline 119
Phosphatidylserines 120
  higher levels of 121
Phosphohistone H3 184, 185
Phosphorylation 201
Photochemotherapy 193
Photodynamic therapy 17, 46, 68-70, 72, 73, 95, 146
Photosensitizers 46
Phototoxicity 4, 144
Phylotype
  determination 132
  in acne 130
Phylum level 164
Physicians Global Assessment 33
Pilosebaceous follicle 90, 200
Pilosebaceous glands
  chronic disorder of 161
  common disorder of 63
Pilosebaceous units 152, 168, 163, 169
Placebo 57
Plant extracts, effect of 90
Plasma exeresis 161
Plasma inflammatory markers 180
  levels of 180, 181
Plasma insulin-like growth factor-1, levels 127
Platelet-derived growth factor 65
Platelet-rich plasma
  efficacy of 64
  treatment 65
Pogostemon patchouli Benth 191
Polyacetylenes 91
Polycystic ovarian syndrome 13, 30, 180
Polyketides 121
Polymerase chain reaction 203
Polymeric network 89
Polyphenols 202
Polyunsaturated fatty acids 128
Poor self-attitude 107
Pore index 52

Post inflammatory
  hyperpigmentation 1, 74
Post-acne erythema 137
Postinflammatory
  hyperpigmentation 41, 81, 92
Postprandial hyperinsulinemia 145
Post-traumatic stress disorder 112
Prenol lipids 121
  levels of 120
Presumptive stressful life event scale 109, 110
Proinflammatory cytokines
  IL-12 101
  interleukin 140
  secretion of 129
Proliferating keratinocytes 150
Proliferative markers Ki67 185
Propionibacterium 118, 174, 188, 204
Propionibacterium acnes 20, 37, 51, 52, 58, 61, 62, 70, 86, 115-118, 137, 146, 148, 154, 155, 158-162, 166-171, 187-190, 201, 204
  activities of 148
  colonization of 62
  derived extracellular vesicles 150, 151
  diversity of 158
  major phylotypes of 159
  proliferation of 96, 196
Propionibacterium communities 150
Propionibacterium species 188
Propolis, combination of 38
Protein level induced 115
Proteins 127
Proteobacteria 163, 164
Proteomic analysis 188
Protoporphyrin IX 17, 70
Pruritic acne 76
Pseudofrost 54
Pseudomonas aeruginosa 90
Pseudopelade of Brocq 178
Psoriasis 18
Psoriatic alopecia, characteristic of 178

Psychological
  distress 92
    cause of 49, 182
    morbidity 162
Psychometric tests 14
Psychosomatic
  approach 110
  strategy 110
Pubertal maturation, signs of 88
Puberty 202
Pyogenic arthritis 175
Pythagorean self-awareness intervention 24

Q

Quadrupole time-of-flight mass spectrometry 120
Quality of life 30, 77, 79, 84, 102, 105, 107, 112
Quercetin 91

R

Radiofrequency evoked thermal effect 78
Rapamycin complex-1 145
  signaling 200
Rapid skin re-epithelialization 80
Rat preputial sebocytes, models use 178
Reactive oxygen species 62, 174
Recombinant human basic fibroblast growth factor 79
Red ginseng ethanol extract 117, 118
Reflectance confocal microscopy 122, 196
Retentional lesions 132
Retinoid 84, 93, 108
  induced cheilitis 45
  topical 2, 44, 68
  use of 63, 85
Ribavirin 18
  side effect of 18
Ribotypes, abundant 101
Rosa damascena Mill 191
Rosacea 113
  analysis of 113
Ruminococcaceae genera 153
Rutin 91

S

Saccharolipids 120, 121
Salicylic acid 53, 54, 60
Salmonella typhimurium 90
Sanger sequencing 203
Santalum 191
Santalum austrocaledonicum 191
Santalum species 190, 191
Sarecycline 3, 4, 144
  microbiological profile of 143
  spectrum of 143
Scarring 74, 26
  causing psychological morbidity 167
Sebaceous
  de novo fatty acid synthesis 201
  drought 149
  follicles 185, 202
  glands 132, 129
    cell lines 178, 180
    proteins in 27
    size 176
  lipogenesis 126
    understanding of 178
  markers 178
Sebocyte apoptosis 27
Sebocytes, primary 178
Sebum
  change of 201
  composition 178
    alteration 196
  derived fatty acids 202
  excretion 193
  free fatty acids 128
  hyperproduction 196
  index 52
  production 6, 24, 176
  secretion 171
Selective retinoic acid receptor-gamma 147
Self-injurious behavior 111
Sequel-like scarring 1
Serological agglutination 101
Serum irisin 175
  level of 176, 177
Sex hormone-binding globulin 30, 31
SIG1459 cream 170

Signaling molecules,
    downstream 157
Signaling networks
    communicating 176
Signs of
    hyperandrogenism 195
    sexual precocity 195
Single nucleotide
    polymorphisms 166, 174
Sirolimus 18
Skimmed milk 128
Skin
    areas
        lesion-free 122
        perilesional-free 122
    biopsy 157
    care products 127
    disease, chronic 203
    disorder, chronic 12
    ecology 149
    homeostasis 155
    irritation, incidences of 61
    microbiome, role of 155
    microbiota 189
        characteristics 35
    surface lipids 120
Sodium diet 128
Sofosbuvir 18
Soft drink consumption,
    daily 144
Soluplus
    extrudates 37
    polymer 36
Specific genes, identification
    of 188
Sphingolipids 121
Spironolactone 6, 33, 93
    safety profile of 32
    treatment switching for 5
Split-face trial comparing 47
Staphylococcus 101
Staphylococcus aureus 58, 147, 204
Staphylococcus epidermidis 58, 90, 137, 188, 190, 204
Staphylococcus species 150
Stearoyl-CoA desaturase 176
Sterol lipids 120
Stevens-Johnson syndrome 18, 57
Stinging nettle leaves 90

Stratum corneum 185
Streptococcus mitis 34
Streptococcus pyogenes 204
Streptococcus species 36
Stress 25
    and acne 105
    in severity 105
    management 110
    reducing techniques 105
Sugar intake, measurement of 145
Suicide probability 111
Sulfone
    agents 60
    compound 48
    compound dapsone 118
Superficial infundibular
    keratinous lining 123
Superficial lesions, removal of 54
Surrogate markers 123
Systemic antibiotics 36, 57
Systemic corticosteroids 164

T

Tacrolimus 18
Tanshinone IIA, antibacterial
    activity of 115-116
Taxonomic, classification of 189
Teledermatology 173
Temperature and humidity 192
Tested peptides in vivo 159
Testosterone 145, 201
Tetracycline 3, 6, 9, 85, 143
Thermosetting gel photodynamic
    therapy 69
Tinnitus 4
TNF-alpha gene promoter
    polymorphism 166, 167
Toll-like receptor 169, 204
    role of 130
Total immunostain expression 28
Transepidermal water loss 186
Transfatty acid 128
Transforming growth factor 65
Transgender adolescents 21
    female-to-male 21
Transgenderism 21
Transmission electron
    microscopy 160

Tretinoin 88, 198
    group 108
Trichloroacetic acid 23
    evaluation the efficacy of 45
Trimethoprim-sulfamethoxazole 60
Triterpenes 121
Tumor necrosis factor 27, 166-168

U

Ultra-performance liquid
    chromatography 120
Urtica dioica 90, 91

V

Venous blood samples 171
Vertigo 4
Vesiculobullous reaction 18
Vestibular 4
    side effects 144
Vetiveria zizanioides 191
Virilizing tumors 30
Virulence factors 188
Visual analogue scale 33
Vitamin
    B12 138
    C 145
    D 124
        concentrations 171
        deficiency 171
        in acne vulgaris, role of 124
        levels 124, 125
        receptor 170
    D3
        gene polymorphisms 172
        levels 136
Vivacubes 196

W

Western blot 115
Whole-genome metagenomic
    sequencing 155

X

Xeroderma 18

Z

Zinc 51
Zouboulis syndrome 178

EU GSPR Authorised Reprsentative
Logos Europe, 9 rue Nicolas Poussin
1700, La Rochelle, France
Phone: +33 (0) 6 67 93 73 78
E-mail: contact@logoseurope.eu

www.ingramcontent.com/pod-product-compliance
Ingram Content Group UK Ltd.
Pitfield, Milton Keynes, MK11 3LW, UK
UKHW050456150426

5217IPUK00025B/1717